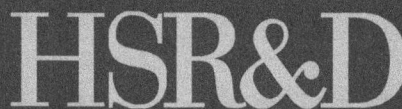

I0470872

Treatment of Anemia in Patients with Heart Disease: A Systematic Review

October 2011

Prepared for:

Department of Veterans Affairs
Veterans Health Administration
Health Services Research & Development Service
Washington, DC 20420

Prepared by:

Evidence-based Synthesis Program (ESP) Center
Portland VA Medical Center
Portland, OR
Devan Kansagara, M.D., M.C.R., Director

Investigators:

Principal Investigator:
Devan Kansagara, M.D., M.C.R.

Co-Investigators:
Edward Dyer, M.D.
Honora Englander, M.D.
David Kagen, M.D.

Research Associate:
Michele Freeman, M.P.H.

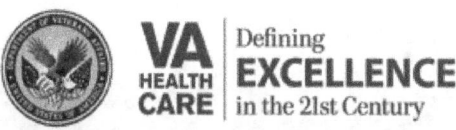

PREFACE

Health Services Research & Development Service's (HSR&D's) Evidence-based Synthesis Program (ESP) was established to provide timely and accurate syntheses of targeted healthcare topics of particular importance to Veterans Affairs (VA) managers and policymakers, as they work to improve the health and healthcare of Veterans. The ESP disseminates these reports throughout VA.

HSR&D provides funding for four ESP Centers and each Center has an active VA affiliation. The ESP Centers generate evidence syntheses on important clinical practice topics, and these reports help:

- develop clinical policies informed by evidence,
- guide the implementation of effective services to improve patient outcomes and to support VA clinical practice guidelines and performance measures, and
- set the direction for future research to address gaps in clinical knowledge.

In 2009, the ESP Coordinating Center was created to expand the capacity of HSR&D Central Office and the four ESP sites by developing and maintaining program processes. In addition, the Center established a Steering Committee comprised of HSR&D field-based investigators, VA Patient Care Services, Office of Quality and Performance, and Veterans Integrated Service Networks (VISN) Clinical Management Officers. The Steering Committee provides program oversight, guides strategic planning, coordinates dissemination activities, and develops collaborations with VA leadership to identify new ESP topics of importance to Veterans and the VA healthcare system.

Comments on this evidence report are welcome and can be sent to Nicole Floyd, ESP Coordinating Center Program Manager, at nicole.floyd@va.gov.

Recommended citation: Kansagara D, Dyer EAW, Englander H, Freeman M, Kagen D, Treatment of Anemia in Patients with Heart Disease: A Systematic Review. VA-ESP Project #05-225; 2011.

This report is based on research conducted by the Evidence-based Synthesis Program (ESP) Center located at the Portland VA Medical Center, Portland OR funded by the Department of Veterans Affairs, Veterans Health Administration, Office of Research and Development, Health Services Research and Development. The findings and conclusions in this document are those of the author(s) who are responsible for its contents; the findings and conclusions do not necessarily represent the views of the Department of Veterans Affairs or the United States government. Therefore, no statement in this article should be construed as an official position of the Department of Veterans Affairs. No investigators have any affiliations or financial involvement (e.g., employment, consultancies, honoraria, stock ownership or options, expert testimony, grants or patents received or pending, or royalties) that conflict with material presented in the report.

TABLE OF CONTENTS

TABLES

FIGURES

EXECUTIVE SUMMARY

BACKGROUND

Anemia is very common in congestive heart failure (CHF) and coronary heart disease (CHD) patients. Anemia in CHF and CHD patients is associated with poorer outcomes, including an increased risk of hospitalization, decreased exercise capacity, and poor quality of life. Despite the association with poorer outcomes, it is unclear whether treating anemia or iron deficiency will improve outcomes. Anemia treatment strategies in heart failure and CHD patients include erythropoiesis-stimulating agents (ESAs) and red blood cell transfusions. Iron replacement in iron deficient patients with or without anemia has also been investigated. The objective of this evidence review is to evaluate the balance of benefit and harms of these treatments. We conducted a systematic review to address the following key questions:

In patients with CHF or CHD,

Key Question #1. What are the health outcome benefits and harms of treating anemia with ESAs?

Key Question #2. What are the health outcome benefits and harms of using iron to treat iron deficiency with or without anemia?

Key Question #3. What are the health outcome benefits and harms of treating anemia with red blood cell transfusions?

METHODS

We conducted searches in Medline® and the Cochrane database of systematic reviews of literature published from 1947 to November 2010, and obtained additional articles from systematic reviews, reference lists of pertinent studies, reviews, editorials, and by consulting experts. We also searched for information about unpublished studies on ClinicalTrials.gov and by contacting pharmaceutical companies directly. Reviewers trained in the critical analysis of literature assessed for relevance the abstracts of citations identified from literatures searches. Full-text articles of potentially relevant abstracts were retrieved for further review. We assessed the internal validity of each study using the Cochrane Risk of Bias tool. We assessed the overall quality of the body of evidence for each outcome by considering the consistency, coherence, and applicability across studies, as well as the internal validity of individual studies, using a method developed by the Grades of Recommendation, Assessment, Development, and Evaluation (GRADE) Working Group. We performed meta-analyses of the effects of ESAs on health outcomes and we conducted additional analyses according to study quality, and according to baseline and change in hemoglobin. We qualitatively reviewed the much smaller number of trials evaluating iron and blood transfusion effects.

RESULTS

We reviewed 1,546 titles and abstracts from the electronic search, and identified an additional 83 from reviewing reference lists, and performing manual searches for recently published studies, and unpublished or ongoing studies.

After applying inclusion/exclusion criteria at the abstract level, 320 full-text articles were reviewed. Of the full-text articles, we rejected 266 that did not meet our inclusion criteria.

ESAs

Sixteen randomized, controlled trials evaluated the impact of ESAs in patients with heart disease. Most of these studies included patients with CHF and reduced systolic function. Though the group of studies as a whole showed ESA use may improve exercise tolerance, this benefit diminished substantially when we included only trials with low risk of bias. Overall, we found little good quality evidence that ESA use consistently improves health outcomes. Some studies found ESA use improved exercise tolerance and duration, but this body of evidence is limited by inconsistency of findings and important methodologic weaknesses. The potential benefits of ESA use seen in some studies may be further tempered by the finding that ESA use is associated with serious harms such as mortality and vascular thrombosis, especially in patients with comorbid chronic kidney disease.

Iron

Two small and one large, well-conducted multicenter trials show that IV iron can improve short-term exercise tolerance and quality of life in patients with symptomatic systolic heart failure and iron deficiency, with or without anemia. The impact on distal health outcomes such as mortality and cardiovascular events remains undertested, as do the long-term effects of such treatment. The evidence supporting symptomatic benefit most closely applies to patients with NYHA III heart failure and evidence of low iron stores.

Blood Transfusions

Nine controlled trials have compared outcomes with the use of a restrictive versus more liberal strategy of red blood cell transfusion among patients with heart disease. In each, conservative use of blood products, guided by a transfusion trigger of hemoglobin 7-9 g/dL, was found to be as safe as transfusion to a higher hemoglobin threshold (most often 10 g/dL). However, the large majority of these studies were quite small, substantially underpowered for detecting important differences in clinical outcomes, and most were conducted in the perioperative setting. Nevertheless, the consistency of the results in the perioperative setting suggests conservative use of transfusion should be the default strategy.

Twenty-one additional observational studies have examined transfusion in patients undergoing percutaneous coronary intervention (PCI) or admitted with acute coronary syndrome, myocardial infarction, or decompensated heart failure. Inconsistency of findings and methodological weaknesses complicate the interpretation of results, but several themes emerge: 1) the evidence strongly suggests that transfusion has no benefit and may be harmful in patients with heart disease and hemoglobin >10 g/dL; 2) outcomes do not appear to improve with transfusion in non-ST-elevation ACS patients with hemoglobin levels down to the 8-9 g/dL range; 3) transfusion is consistently associated with higher mortality risk in the unselected PCI population, across multiple studies with mean nadir hemoglobin of 8-9 g/dL; and 4) the elevated risk in the PCI population is seen in patients with anemia related or unrelated to bleeding but may be higher in the non-bleeding anemic population. There is no evidence to guide decision-making in the stable coronary disease population, and the two studies in decompensated heart failure have conflicting results.

DISCUSSION/CONCLUSION

Anemia commonly complicates heart disease. Despite its association with poor outcomes and a biologically plausible argument supporting anemia correction, we found little evidence that use of erythropoiesis-stimulating agents or blood transfusions improves health outcomes in patients with heart disease. A limited evidence base consisting mainly of one trial suggests correction of iron deficiency in patients with symptomatic heart failure improves exercise tolerance and quality of life. The application of the evidence to different patient subsets is described in the main report and is summarized in the following table.

EXECUTIVE SUMMARY TABLE

Summary of the evidence for the effects of ESAs, iron and blood transfusions for anemia, by patient population and outcome

Treatment	Outcome	Effect*	GRADE Classification†	Comment
Stable CHF, and no worse than stage 3 CKD				
ESAs	Exercise tolerance and duration	(~)	Moderate	Inconsistent results and methodologic weaknesses in some studies limit the evidence base. Overall, studies with low risk of bias found no significant effect.
	Quality of life	(~)	Low	Infrequent reporting, inconsistent results, the variety of instruments used, and methodologic weaknesses in some studies greatly limit the evidence base.
	Mortality	(~)	Low	Based on mainly small, single center trials with limited power and low event rates.
	Hospitalizations	(~)	Low	Inconsistent results and methodologic weaknesses in some studies limit the evidence base. The two studies with low risk of bias found no significant effect.
	Harms including hypertension, cerebrovascular and thrombotic events	(~)	Low	Based on mainly small, single center trials with low event rates.
Iron	Exercise tolerance and duration	(+)	Moderate/High	One well-conducted large multicenter trial and two smaller trials found benefit.
	Quality of life	(+)	Moderate/High	One well-conducted large multicenter trial and two smaller trials found benefit.
	Mortality	(~)/(+)	Low	The one large trial showed a trend towards benefit, but was, like the two smaller trials, not powered for this outcome.
	Cardiovascular events	(+)	Moderate	One large multicenter trial found benefit, but follow-up was relatively short.
	Serious harms	(~)	Moderate	Based on one large and two small trials.
Blood transfusions	All outcomes	(0)		No evidence.

Treatment	Outcome	Effect*	GRADE Classification†	Comment
Stable CHF, and stage 4 or 5 CKD				
ESAs	Exercise tolerance and duration	(0)		No evidence. Trials including subgroups of CHF patients did not report this outcome separately.
	Quality of life	(~)	Low	One large trial of heart disease patients including large subgroup of CHF patients, but subgroup specific data not available.
	Mortality	(–)	Moderate	Based on two large trials including large numbers with CHF; in one trial the increased risk of mortality was not significant; type and severity of CHF not reported.
	Cardiovascular events	(~)	High	Based on three large trials including large numbers with CHF; type and severity of CHF not reported.
	Venous thrombosis	(–)	Moderate	Based on two large trials including large numbers with CHF; type and severity of CHF not reported; effects of more moderate hemoglobin targets not tested.
	Hypertension, cerebrovascular events	(–)	Low	Based on one large trial including large numbers with CHF, but CHF subgroup data not separately reported for this outcome.
Iron	All outcomes	(0)		No evidence.
Blood transfusions	All outcomes	(0)		No evidence.
Decompensated CHF				
ESAs	All outcomes	(0)		No evidence.
Iron	All outcomes	(0)		No evidence.
Blood transfusions	Mortality	(–)	Very low	Two observational studies found conflicting results – one showed harm, one a possible benefit.
Stable CHD				
ESAs	Mortality	(–)	Low	One large trial of heart disease patients including large subgroup of CHD patients, but subgroup specific data not available. Patients with ESRD, unclear application to other populations.
	Quality of life	(~)	Low	One large trial of heart disease patients including large subgroup of CHD patients, but subgroup specific data not available. Patients with ESRD, unclear application to other populations.
	Venous thrombosis	(–)	Low	One large trial of heart disease patients including large subgroup of CHD patients, but subgroup specific data not available. Patients with ESRD, unclear application to other populations.
	All other outcomes	(0)		No evidence.
Iron	All outcomes	(0)		No evidence.

Treatment	Outcome	Effect*	GRADE Classification†	Comment
Blood transfusions	All outcomes	(0)		No evidence.
Acute coronary syndrome				
ESAs	All outcomes	(0)		No evidence.
Iron	All outcomes	(0)		No evidence.
Blood transfusions	Mortality	(~)	Moderate	Two RCTs, one with limited applicability to non ICU population, showed no benefit from transfusing above Hgb > 10 g/dL. Observational studies in PCI patients consistently showed no benefit and possible harm.
	Cardiovascular events	(~)	Low	Two RCTs found conflicting results: one found harm, a larger trial found no effect. Observational studies did not commonly report this as a separate outcome.
Non-cardiac surgery				
ESAs	All outcomes	(0)		No evidence.
Iron	All outcomes	(0)		No evidence.
Blood transfusions	Mortality	(~)	Low	One large RCT, but reported only in abstract form and only applicable to hip fracture patients.
Cardiac surgery				
ESAs	All outcomes	(0)		No evidence.
Iron	All outcomes	(0)		No evidence.
Blood transfusions	Mortality	(~)	Moderate	Two large and two small RCTs with some methodologic weaknesses.

GRADE = Grades of Recommendation, Assessment, Development, and Evaluation; ICU = intensive care unit; RCT = randomized controlled trial.

* Effect: (+) benefit; (–) harm; (~) mixed findings/no effect; (0) no evidence.

† GRADE classification: high = further research is very unlikely to change our confidence on the estimate of effect; moderate = further research is likely to have an important impact on our confidence in the estimate of effect and may change the estimate; low = further research is very likely to have an important impact on our confidence in the estimate of effect and is likely to change the estimate; very low = any estimate of effect is very uncertain.

EVIDENCE REPORT

INTRODUCTION

Anemia is very common in patients with heart disease: about one-third of congestive heart failure (CHF) patients and 10 to 20 percent of coronary heart disease (CHD) patients are anemic, though prevalence estimates vary according to the definition used and illness burden in the population being studied.[1-3] The etiology of anemia in heart disease remains incompletely understood, though there are a number of factors that likely contribute including: comorbid chronic kidney disease, blunted erythropoietin production, hemodilution, aspirin-induced gastrointestinal blood loss, the use of renin-angiotensin-aldosterone system (RAAS) blockers, cytokine-mediated inflammation (anemia of chronic disease), and gut malabsorption with consequent nutritional deficiency. Iron deficiency is also common. Cytokine mediated sequestration of iron in the reticuloendothelial system may contribute to a functional iron deficiency, while an absolute deficiency can result from decreased oral iron absorption associated with cytokine induced hepcidin synthesis.[4]

Anemia is associated with poor outcomes in patients with heart disease, but it is unclear whether anemia directly and independently contributes to these poor outcomes, or whether it simply reflects more severe underlying illness and comorbidities.[5-7] Strategies to correct anemia and/or iron deficiency have included erythropoiesis-stimulating agents, iron supplementation, and red blood cell transfusions. The purpose of this systematic review is to summarize the health outcome effects of each of these treatment strategies in adult medicine patients with heart disease.

METHODS

TOPIC DEVELOPMENT

The review was commissioned by the Department of Veterans Affairs' Evidence-based Synthesis Program. We conferred with VA and non-VA experts to select the patients and subgroups, interventions, outcomes, and setting addressed in the review. We addressed the following key questions in our review of the literature:

In patients with CHF or CHD,

Key Question 1. What are the health outcome benefits and harms of treating anemia with erythropoiesis-stimulating agents (ESAs)?

Key Question #2. What are the health outcome benefits and harms of using iron to treat iron deficiency with or without anemia?

Key Question #3. What are the health outcome benefits and harms of treating anemia with red blood cell transfusions?

The criteria for patient population, treatment and comparator interventions, outcomes of interest, and patient care setting are outlined below:

Patients: Adult patients with symptomatic CHF (with or without reduced systolic function) or CHD (acute coronary syndrome, post-acute coronary syndrome, history of MI or angina,) and anemia or iron deficiency.

Interventions:

- ESAs with or without iron: These include erythropoietin and darbepoeitin

- Iron: Intravenous or oral

- Red blood cell transfusion

Comparator: Usual care, placebo

Outcomes: Mortality (all-cause and disease specific), hospitalization (all-cause and disease-specific), exercise tolerance or duration (any metric, most commonly NYHA class, 6 minute walk test), quality of life, cardiovascular events (myocardial infarction, heart failure exacerbation, need for revascularization)

Setting: Inpatient or outpatient

Figure 1 illustrates the analytic framework that guided our review and synthesis.

Figure 1. Analytic Framework

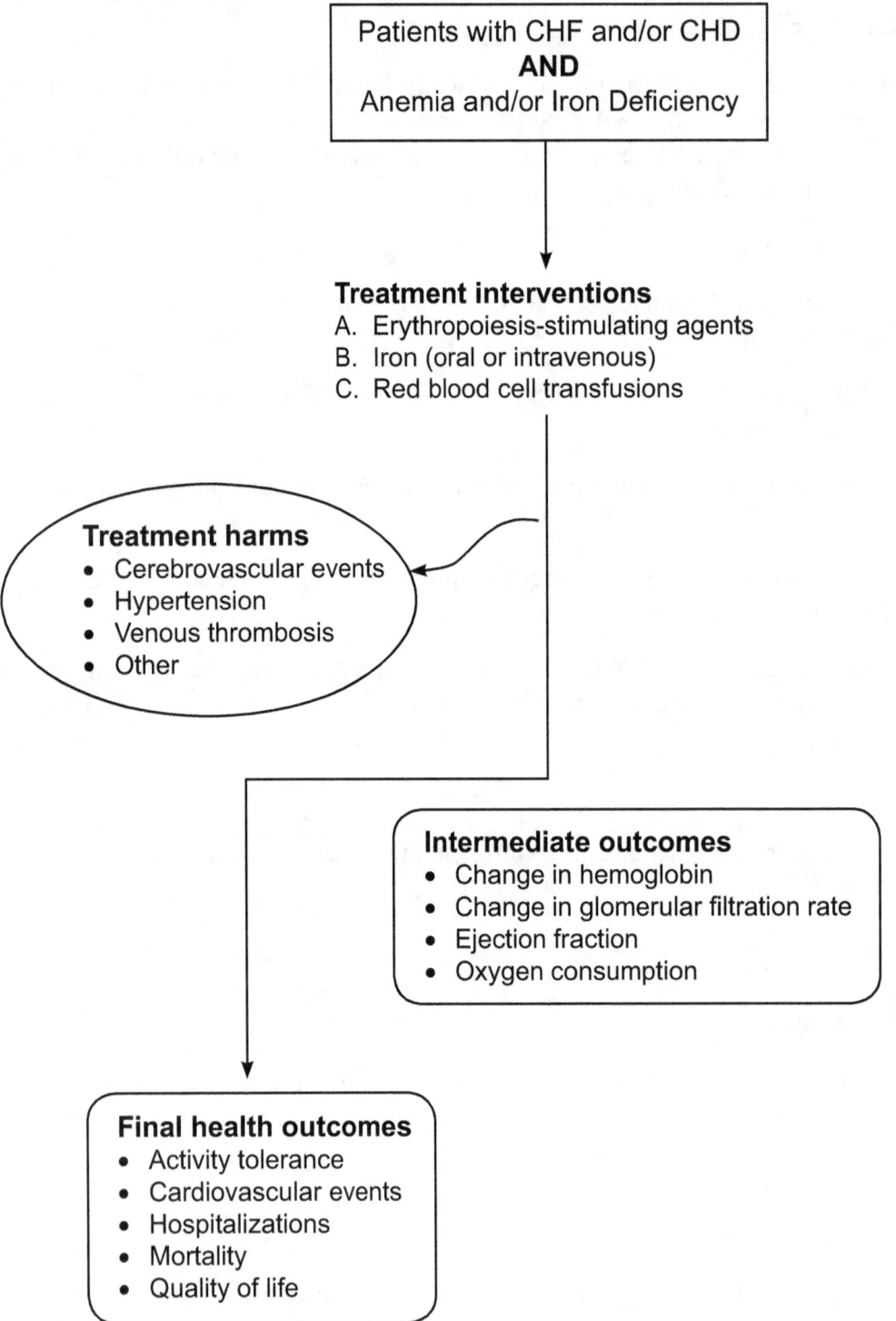

SEARCH STRATEGY

We conducted a search in Medline® and the Cochrane database of systematic reviews of literature published from 1947 to November 2010. Appendix A provides the search strategy in detail. We obtained additional articles from systematic reviews, reference lists of pertinent studies, reviews, editorials, and by consulting experts. We also searched for information about unpublished studies on ClinicalTrials.gov. All citations were imported into an electronic database (EndNote X1).

STUDY SELECTION

Three reviewers assessed for relevance the abstracts of citations identified from literature searches. Two reviewers independently assessed for inclusion full-text articles of potentially relevant abstracts based on the eligibility criteria shown in Appendix B. Disagreements were resolved through a consensus process.

Eligible articles had English-language abstracts and provided primary data relevant to the key questions. We included studies of anemic patients (hemoglobin < 13 g/dL in men, < 12 g/dL in women) with symptomatic CHF (with or without reduced systolic function), CHD (acute coronary syndrome, post-acute coronary syndrome, history of MI or angina), or both. Further eligibility criteria varied depending on the question of interest, as described below.

To evaluate the efficacy of ESAs, we considered prospective, controlled clinical trials of ESAs compared either to placebo or to less intensive ESA use in patients with anemia and heart disease. In evaluating the efficacy of iron, we included studies with mixed populations of anemic and non-anemic patients, but then described how treatment effects might differ for anemic and non-anemic patients. We did include studies of broader patient populations as long as they separately reported outcomes data for the subpopulation of patients with heart disease.

Included studies had to report at least one prespecified patient-centered health outcome which we defined as clinically important outcomes apparent to the patient (Appendix B). We excluded studies reporting only intermediate physiologic outcomes such as change in ejection fraction or oxygen delivery metrics.

Based on an initial exploratory search of red blood cell transfusions in patients with heart disease, we recognized there was a dearth of controlled clinical trial data and that current recommendations for blood transfusion use in heart disease patients are largely based on interpretation of observational studies. Therefore, to better understand the evidence currently guiding clinical practice, we included observational studies as well as controlled clinical trials that reported at least one of the above listed health outcomes. Given the complex technique of cardiac surgery, involving induction of hypothermia, cardioplegia, and establishment of an extracorporeal circuit, we felt that the potential confounding factors were too vast to permit use of observational data to guide decision-making. Therefore, for this population, we elected to consider controlled trials only.

To evaluate the harms of ESAs, iron, and blood transfusion, we collected adverse events data from all the included trials, and we specifically gathered data on the following events from each trial: hypertension, venous thromboembolic events (including deep venous thrombosis, pulmonary embolism, and vascular access thrombosis), and ischemic cerebrovascular events.

DATA ABSTRACTION

From each study, we abstracted the following: study design, objectives, setting, population characteristics (including sex, age, left ventricular ejection fraction, baseline NYHA class, definition of CHD), subject eligibility and exclusion criteria, number of subjects, years of enrollment, duration of follow-up, the study and comparator interventions (including route and dosage), important co-interventions (i.e., iron administration in ESA studies), baseline hemoglobin, change in hemoglobin, health outcomes, and adverse events.

STUDY QUALITY

Two reviewers independently assessed the quality of each trial using a tool developed by the Cochrane Collaboration.[8] Disagreements were resolved through discussion. This tool asks the following questions about the methodologic characteristics of each study to guide assessment of the risk of bias:

- Was the allocation sequence adequately generated?
- Was allocation adequately concealed?
- Blinding of participants, personnel and outcome assessors: Was knowledge of the allocated intervention adequately prevented during the study?
- Were incomplete outcome data adequately addressed?
- Are reports of the study free of suggestion of selective outcome reporting?
- Was the study apparently free of other problems that could put it at a high risk of bias? (We assessed whether or not there were extreme baseline differences between groups.)

Each study was then given an overall summary assessment of either low, high, or unclear risk of bias. The risk of bias within a given study can vary according to outcome. For instance, the risk of bias associated with lack of blinding might be low for mortality outcomes, but high for more subjective outcomes such as quality of life or symptom scores.

Though there is no widely accepted standard for quality assessment of observational studies, we used the following questions to guide a comparison of observational study methodologic characteristics:

1. Was the selection of patients for inclusion unbiased? (Was any group of patients systematically excluded?)
2. Was there important differential loss to follow-up or overall high loss to follow-up? (Numbers should be given for each group.)
3. Were the events investigated specified and defined?
4. Was there a clear description of the techniques used to identify the events?
5. Was there unbiased and accurate ascertainment of events (that is, by independent ascertainers using a validated ascertainment technique)?
6. Were potential confounding variables and risk factors identified and examined using acceptable statistical techniques?
7. Was the duration of follow-up reasonable for investigated events?

Within question 6, we specifically assessed whether each study: 1) conducted an analysis adjusting for patient propensity to receive a blood transfusion, 2) accounted for bleeding complications – whether procedurally related or not – in the study population, and 3) accounted for the timing of transfusion given the potential for issues such as survival bias in which patients who died could not have received a transfusion.

We do not report an overall summary assessment for observational studies because there are no validated criteria for doing so and all would be poorly valid in determining the health outcome effects of blood transfusions.

Appendix C provides the details of our quality assessment of trials and observational studies.

RATING THE BODY OF EVIDENCE

We assessed the overall quality of evidence for outcomes using a method developed by the GRADE Working Group.[9] The GRADE method considers the consistency, coherence, and applicability of a body of evidence, as well as the internal validity of individual studies, to classify the grade of evidence across outcomes as follows:

- High = Further research is very unlikely to change our confidence on the estimate of effect.
- Moderate = Further research is likely to have an important impact on our confidence in the estimate of effect and may change the estimate.
- Low = Further research is very likely to have an important impact on our confidence in the estimate of effect and is likely to change the estimate.
- Very Low = Any estimate of effect is very uncertain.

DATA SYNTHESIS

We performed meta-analyses of ESA trials for each of the following outcomes: mean difference in the change of NYHA class, exercise duration during the six-minute walk test, all-cause mortality, hospitalizations, cardiovascular events, hypertension events, and ischemic cerebrovascular events. We abstracted the number of events and total subjects from each treatment arm, and obtained a pooled estimate of relative risk (RR) using a random effects model.[10] We did not meta-analyze quality of life outcomes because we felt a quantitative summary estimate of effect would be less meaningful than a descriptive approach given the variety of assessment tools used.

In order to determine the influence study quality may have had on summary results, we ran analyses for all outcomes excluding those studies with high or unclear risk of bias. To determine whether the effects of ESAs were modified by anemia characteristics, we conducted analyses according to baseline hemoglobin and mean change in hemoglobin in the intervention group, using 11g/dL and 2 g/dL, respectively, as the cutpoints based on distribution of values among included studies. If only the hematocrit was reported, we used a conversion of 3:1 to approximate the hemoglobin value.

Statistical heterogeneity was assessed by Cochran's Q test and I^2 statistic.[8] Because of the small number of trials that could be combined, we did not perform assessments for publication bias.[11] All analyses were performed using Stata 10.0 (StataCorp, College Station, TX, 2007).

Because there were only three trials examining the effects of iron therapy, with one large trial dominating results, we decided to only qualitatively synthesize these results. We also qualitatively synthesized the mostly observational blood transfusion literature.

PEER REVIEW

A draft version of this report was sent to the technical expert panel and additional peer reviewers. The comments and suggestions we received from reviewers and our responses in revising the report are provided in Appendix D.

RESULTS

LITERATURE FLOW

We reviewed 1,546 titles and abstracts from the electronic search, and identified an additional 83 from reviewing reference lists, and performing manual searches for recently published studies, and unpublished or ongoing studies.

After applying inclusion/exclusion criteria at the abstract level, 320 full-text articles were reviewed, as shown in Figure 2. Of the full-text articles, we rejected 266 that did not meet our inclusion criteria.

Figure 2. Literature Flow – Anemia and CHF

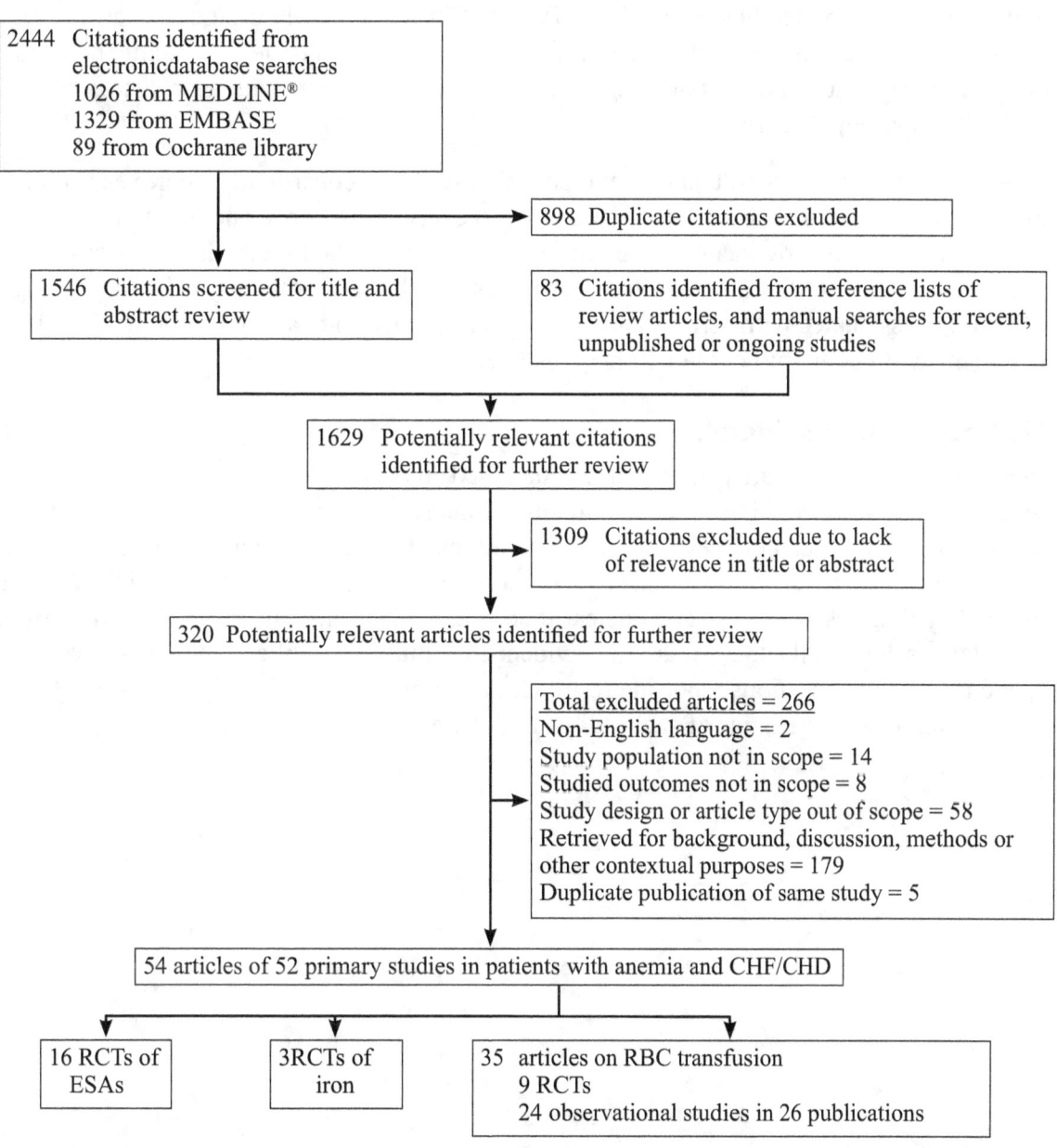

KEY QUESTION #1. In patients with CHF or CHD, what are the health outcome benefits and harms of treating anemia with ESAs?

Summary

Sixteen randomized, controlled trials evaluated the impact of ESAs in patients with heart disease (Table 1).[12-27] We excluded one study[28] whose patient population was included in a subsequent publication.[21, 28] Eleven trials enrolled patients with CHF, and in the 10 trials reporting systolic function, the mean ejection fraction was $\leq 35\%$. Most patients had comorbid CHD. Two trials included roughly even proportions of patients with CHD and CHF,[14, 26] and only one trial focused exclusively on patients with CHD.[27] The most commonly reported health outcomes were exercise tolerance measures such as NYHA (nine trials), and exercise duration as measured by the six-minute walk test (five trials) or the Naughton protocol (two trials). Nine trials reported mortality and seven trials reported hospitalizations. Two trials were primarily designed to assess the comparative effects of ESAs titrated to high or low hemoglobin targets in anemic patients with chronic kidney disease, but included a large proportion of patients with heart disease for whom adequate subgroup data are reported.[13, 14]

Overall, we found little good quality evidence that ESA use consistently improves health outcomes. Some studies found ESA use improved exercise tolerance and duration, but this body of evidence is limited by inconsistency of findings and important methodologic weaknesses. The potential benefits of ESA use seen in some studies may be further tempered by the finding that ESA use is associated with serious harms such as mortality and vascular thrombosis, especially in patients with comorbid chronic kidney disease.

Methodologic Considerations

We characterized the quality of each of the included studies according to the impact methodologic flaws could have on an outcome of interest. For example, flaws such as the lack of patient and/or outcome assessor blinding could lead to biased results for subjective outcomes such as exercise tolerance. Five trials contained serious methodologic flaws which could have biased key findings,[12, 15, 21, 24, 25] and unclear reporting made it difficult to assess the risk of bias in one trial.[17] Additionally, there was some evidence for multiple publication bias: in two cases we found multiple publications reporting results for apparently overlapping populations.[16, 18, 21, 28] The methodologic characteristics of each study are detailed in Appendix C, Table 1.

Table 1. Characteristics of randomized controlled trials of ESA therapy in patients with CHF or CHD

Study ID Setting Months of follow-up	N (T v C); Demographics: % male; % race/ethnicity; mean age (yr)	Clinical subgroup (CHF/CAD); Mean LVEF %; % on RAAS blockers (T v C)	Baseline kidney function, GFR or Serum Cr (T v C)	Intervention (Drug, Dose) v Control	Baseline measures of iron stores (T v C)	Iron in Tx group	Iron in Control group	Baseline Hgb (T v C)	Mean change in Hgb (T v C)	Funding source
Studies conducted in patients with CHF										
Comin-Colet, 2009[12] Single-center Spain 15.3 months	N: 27 v 38 male: 70.4 v 50.0 mean age: 74 v 74	Advanced CHF + CRI: LVEF: 34.5 v 34.6 NYHA II: 66.7 v 81.6 NYHA IV: 33.3 v 18.4 Ischemic etiology: 66.7 v 55.3 ACEI/ARB: 70.4 v 76.3 Aldo antag: 74.1 v 60.5	GFR: 48.1 v 50.3	Epoetin 4000u IV weekly, adjusted to target Hgb 12.5-14.5 + iron sucrose IV 200mg weekly x 5-6 wks to target ferritin>400, then q 4-6 wks. Control group was not given a placebo.	ferritin: 220.7 v 140.7 TSAT%: 23.2 v 19.9	Y	N	10.9 v 10.9	1.7 v 0.4	NR
Ghali, 2008[19] STAMINA-HeFT Multicenter (65), phase 2 study 12 months; most endpoints at 6 months	N: 162 v 157 male: 57 v 68 white: 77 v 85 black: 14 v 11 mean age: 68 v 69	LVEF: 35 v 36. NYHA I: 1 v 2 NYHA II: 38 v 32 NYHA III: 59 v 62 NYHA IV: 2 v 3 RAAS blockers: 90 v 90	GFR: 47.2 v 47.5	Darbepoeitin alfa 0.75mcg/kg sc q 2 wks titrated to target Hgb ~ 14 vs. "matching placebo"	ferritin: 121 v 124 TSAT%: 23.5 v 23.5	Y, daily elemental oral iron	Y, daily elemental oral iron	11.5 v 11.3	Median Hgb change at 27 weeks: 1.8 v 0.3 53 weeks: 2.1 v 0.5	Amgen
Kourea, 2008[17] Single-center Greece 3 months	N: 21 v 20 male: 76 v 75 mean age: 73 v 65	LVEF: 2 v 8 NYHA II: 38 v 45 NYHA III: 62 v 55 Ischemic CM: 62 v 60 ACEI: 71 v 65 ARE: 19 v 20 Aldo artag: 57 v 55	Cr: 1.7 v 1.7	Darbepoeitin alfa 1.5 mcg/kg sc q 20 days titrated to target Hgb ~ 14 vs. 0.9% saline	ferritin: 144 v 159 Iron: 45 v 59	Y, oral iron 250 mg BID	Y, oral iron 250 mg BID	10.9 v 11.4	1.6 v -0.9	none
Mancini, 2003[24] Single center US 3 months	N: 15 v 8 male: 86.7 v 62.5 race/ethnicity NR mean age: 60 v 55	NYHA 3-4 LVEF: 24 v 21 h/o CAD: 53.3 v 50 RAAS blockers not different between both groups; most were on RAAS blockers (NOS)	Cr: 1.6 v 1.6	Epoetin 5000 sc TIW - titrated up to 10,000 TIW if Hgb did not increase 1 g/dL vs. saline	NR	Y, oral iron 325 mg daily	N	10.9 v 11.0	3.3 v 0.6 (T increased from 11 to 14.3 and C 10.9 to 11.5)	NIH
Palazzuoli, 2007[21] Single-center Italy 12 months	N: 26 v 25 male: 58 v 64 mean age: 74 v 72	LFEF: 30 v 31 NYHA III: 69 v 68 NYHA IV: 30.8 v 32 Mean NYHA: 3.4 v 3.6 ACEI: 69 v 64 ARE: 19 v 28	GFR: 43 v 45	Beta erythropoeitin 6000 IU sc twice weekly to goal Hgb 12-12.5 vs. saline	NR	Y, oral iron gluconate 300 mg daily	Y, oral iron gluconate 300 mg daily	10.4 +/- 0.6 v 10.6 +/- 0.7	2.0 v -0.1	none

Treatment of Anemia in Patients with Heart Disease: A Systematic Review

Study ID Setting Months of follow-up	N (T v C); Demographics: % male; % race/ethnicity; mean age (yr)	Clinical subgroup (CHF/CAD); Mean LVEF %; % on RAAS blockers (T v C)	Baseline kidney function, GFR or Serum Cr (T v C)	Intervention (Drug, Dose) v Control	Baseline measures of iron stores (T v C)	Iron in Tx group	Iron in Control group	Baseline Hgb (T v C)	Mean change in Hgb (T v C)	Funding source
Palazzuoli, 2009[15] Single-center Italy 12 months	N: 26 v 25 No demographic information reported	LVEF 30.1 vs 30.8 RAAS blockers NR	Cr: 2.3 vs 2.4	Epoetin 6000 sc BIW vs. saline placebo for first four months	NR	FeGluconate 300 mg QD	FeGluconate 300 mg QD	9.6 v 9.3	Final Hgb: 12.4 v 10.4	NR
Parissis, 2008[18] Single center Greece 3 months	N: 21 v 11 mean age: 72 v 69	LVEF: 26 v 28 NYHA II: 19 v 27 NYHA III: 81 v 73 Ischemic related: 90 v 82 ACEI: 71 v 73 ARB 19 v 18 Aldo antag: 57 v 55	Cr: 1.7 v 1.8	Darbepoeitin alfa 1.5mcg/kg sc q 20 days vs. 0.9% saline	ferritin: 153 +/- 119 v 170 +/- 135.	Y, oral iron sulfate 125 mg BID	Y, oral iron sulfate 125 mg BID	11.0 v 11.4	Final Hgb: 12.8 v 11.8	NR
Parissis, 2009[16] Single center Greece 3 months	N: 15 v 15 mean age: 71 v 67 male: 73.3 v 66.7	LVEF: 28 v 27 NYHA II: 53.3 v 60 NYHA III: 46.7 v 40 Ischemic: 86.7 v 73.3 ACEI: 93.3 v 86.7 ARB: 6.7 v 2/15	Cr: 1.6 v 1.5	Darbepoeitin alfa 1.5 mcg/kg q 20 days vs. 0.9% saline	ferritin: 133 +/- 126 v 127 +/- 112.	Y, oral iron sulfate 125 mg BID	Y, oral iron sulfate 125 mg BID	11.2 v 11.5	1.6 v 0.4	none
Ponikowski, 2007[23] Multicenter 6 months (27 weeks)	N: 19 v 22 male: 63 v 45 white: 95 v 100 asian: 5 v 0 mean age: 72 v 70	NYHA I: 0 v 5 NYHA II: 58 v 36 NYHA III: 42 v 59 Ischemic: 84 v 86 RAAS blockers NR	GFR: 59 v 52	Darbepoeitin alfa 0.75mcg/ kg sc q 2 wks, titrated to Hgb 13-15 vs. placebo "in identical single-dose vials"	median ferritin (25th and 75th): 71 (46, 143) v 161 (83, 256). TSAT%: 25.3 (SD 6.6) v 34.6 (SD 12.8).	N, not specified	N, not specified	11.8 v 11.6	2.4 v 0.9	Amgen
Silverberg, 2001[25] Single center Israel 12.4 ± 8.2 months	N: 16 v 16 mean age: 75.3 v 72.2 male: 69 v 75	LVEF: 30.8 v 28.4 Mean NYHA: 3.8 v 3.5 Ischemic: 69 v 62.5 ACEI: 87.5 v 87.5 ARB: 6.6 v 12.5	Cr: 1.7 v 1.4	Erythropoietin 4000 IU sc weekly adjusted to goal Hgb 12.5 Control not reported.	ferritin: 221 (SD 165) v 264 (SD 162), NS. TSAT%: 25.1 (SD 12.9) v 22.5 (SD 16.7), NS.	Y, IV ferric sucrose 200 mg q 2 weeks	N	10.3 v 10.9	2.6 v -0.1	none
Van Veldhuisen, 2007[22] Multi-center (44 sites, 15 countries) 6 months	N: 110 v 55 male: 56 v 62 white: 93 v 89 black: 5 v 7 asian: 3 v 4 mean age: 71 v 71	LVEF: 29 v 27 NYHA I: 3 v 2 NYHA II: 36 v 44 NYHA III: 59 v 53 NYHA IV: 2 v 2 Ischemic: 69 v 64 ACEI: 77 v 75 ARB: 18 v 20 ACE/ARB: 94 v 91	GFR: 56.5 v 53.5	Darbepoeitin alpha 0.75 mcg/ kg sc q 2 wks OR 50 mcg (fixed dose) vs. identical placebo provided by Amgen	ferritin: 198 (SD 232) v 200 (SD 224). TSAT%: 26 (SD 9) v 25 (SD 8).	Y, 200 mg oral iron daily	Y, 200 mg oral iron daily	11.5 v 11.4	1.87 (0.75 mcg/kg) v 0.07	Amgen

Study ID Setting Months of follow-up	N (T v C); Demographics: % male; % race/ethnicity; mean age (yr)	Clinical subgroup (CHF/CAD); Mean LVEF %; % on RAAS blockers (T v C)	Baseline kidney function, GFR or Serum Cr (T v C)	Intervention (Drug, Dose) v Control	Baseline measures of iron stores (T v C)	Iron in Tx group	Iron in Control group	Baseline Hgb (T v C)	Mean change in Hgb (T v C)	Funding source
Studies conducted in patients with CAD										
Bellinghieri, 1994[27] Single-center Italy 24 months	N: 26 v 10 male: 50 vs. 70 race NR mean age: 62.4 v 64.2	CAD (at east one episode of angina or dysrhythmia in last year) RAAS blockers NR	All pts ESRD on HD	Epoeitin IV 25 IU/kg post each HD Control not reported.	NR	NR	NR	NR in both groups	8.1 to 8.97 in Tx group	NR
Studies conducted in patients with CHF or CAD										
Besarab 1998[26] 2008[20] Multicenter US 30 months	N: 618 v 615 male: 50 v 48 white: 45 v 42 black 41 v 44 Hispanic: 8 v 9 mean age: 65 v 64	CHF (44 v 47) or CHD LVEF NR RAAS blockers: no significant difference between groups (NOS)	All pts ESRD on HD	Epoetin IV or SQ to target Hct 42 ±3 vs. Epoetin IV or SQ to target Hct 30 ± 3	ferritin: 334 v 403 (p = 0.002) TSAT%: 26.8 v 26.3	IV iron dextran in 526/618 pts	IV iron dextran in 464/615 pts	Hct: 30.5 v 30.5	Change in Hct: approx 10 v 0%	Amgen
Studies analyzing a CHF/CAD subgroup of patients with CKD										
Pfeffer, 2009[14] Heart disease subset of TREAT Multi-center, international 29 months	N: 1287 v 1355 (2,636/4,044 enrolled had CVD Hx) male: 46 mean age: 70 white 69 black: 19 Hispanic: 9.3	C'/D: 67.9 CHF: 50.2 PAD: 31.8 RAAS blockers: 77.7	GFR: 34	Darbepoeitin alpha titrated to high (13.0 g/dL) vs. low (9.0 g/dL) Hgb target	TSAT%: 23 ferritin: 134	N	N	10.4	For overall cohort (n=4,044) Median achieved Hgb 12.5 (change of 2.1) v 10.6 (change of 0.1)	Amgen
Szczech, 2010[13] CHF subset of CHOIR 36 months	N: 192 v 183 mean age (Hgb 13.5 group v Hgb 11.3 group): 70.2 v 69.5 male: 46.4 v 56.3 black: 29.3 v 27.3 Hispanic: 9.4 v 12.0	CHF	GFR: 26.9 v 26.0	Epoetin alpha titrated to high (13.5 g/dL) vs. low (11.3 g/dL) Hgb target	ferritin (Hgb 13.5 group vs Hgb 11.3 group): 159.5 v 193.5, p=0.050. TSAT%: 22.1 v 24.1, p=0.043.			Hgb 13.5: 10.0 Hgb 11.3: 10.0		CHOIR funded by Ortho Biotech and Johnson & Johnson. This secondary analysis by NIH.

Exercise Tolerance and Duration

Overall, though there is some data that ESAs may improve exercise tolerance, the body of evidence is limited by inconsistent results and the methodologic weaknesses of some studies. Pooled results from nine trials reporting change in NYHA scores were highly heterogeneous and found a decline in NYHA scores in ESA-treated patients while control patients generally maintained stable scores or worsened (mean difference in NYHA scores treatment vs. control, -0.77, 95% CI -1.21 to -0.32, I^2=96.0%, Figure 3). However, this improvement was significantly attenuated when we limited the analysis to the four methodologically stronger trials (mean difference in NYHA scores -0.15; 95% CI -0.36 to 0.06; I^2=62.1%, Figure 4). The largest of these trials randomized 319 patients to twice-monthly darbepoietin or saline placebo, and measured exercise duration, tolerance and quality of life outcomes at 27 weeks.[19] The authors found darbepoietin had no effect on any of the outcomes despite raising hemoglobin by 1.8 g/dL on average.

Figure 3. Change in NYHA scores in CHF patients: mean difference comparing ESA to control group

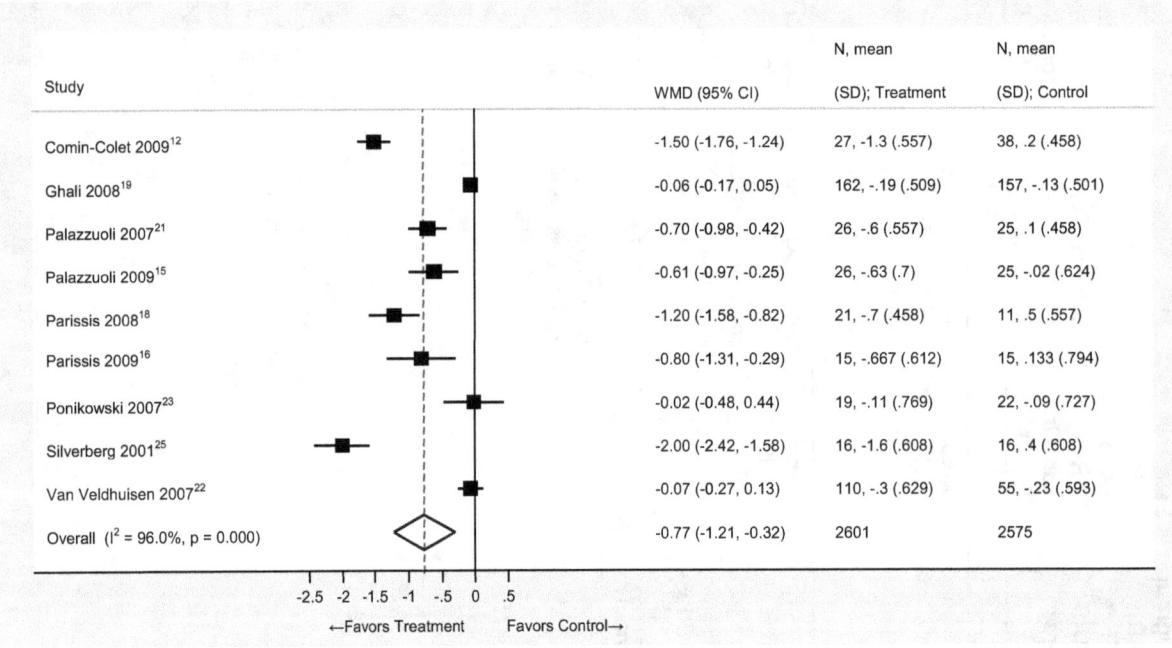

Study	WMD (95% CI)	N, mean (SD); Treatment	N, mean (SD); Control
Comin-Colet 2009[12]	-1.50 (-1.76, -1.24)	27, -1.3 (.557)	38, .2 (.458)
Ghali 2008[19]	-0.06 (-0.17, 0.05)	162, -.19 (.509)	157, -.13 (.501)
Palazzuoli 2007[21]	-0.70 (-0.98, -0.42)	26, -.6 (.557)	25, .1 (.458)
Palazzuoli 2009[15]	-0.61 (-0.97, -0.25)	26, -.63 (.7)	25, -.02 (.624)
Parissis 2008[18]	-1.20 (-1.58, -0.82)	21, -.7 (.458)	11, .5 (.557)
Parissis 2009[16]	-0.80 (-1.31, -0.29)	15, -.667 (.612)	15, .133 (.794)
Ponikowski 2007[23]	-0.02 (-0.48, 0.44)	19, -.11 (.769)	22, -.09 (.727)
Silverberg 2001[25]	-2.00 (-2.42, -1.58)	16, -1.6 (.608)	16, .4 (.608)
Van Veldhuisen 2007[22]	-0.07 (-0.27, 0.13)	110, -.3 (.629)	55, -.23 (.593)
Overall (I^2 = 96.0%, p = 0.000)	-0.77 (-1.21, -0.32)	2601	2575

←Favors Treatment   Favors Control→

Figure 4. Change in NYHA scores in CHF patients – studies with low risk of bias, and excluding studies with duplicate patient populations: mean difference comparing ESA to control group

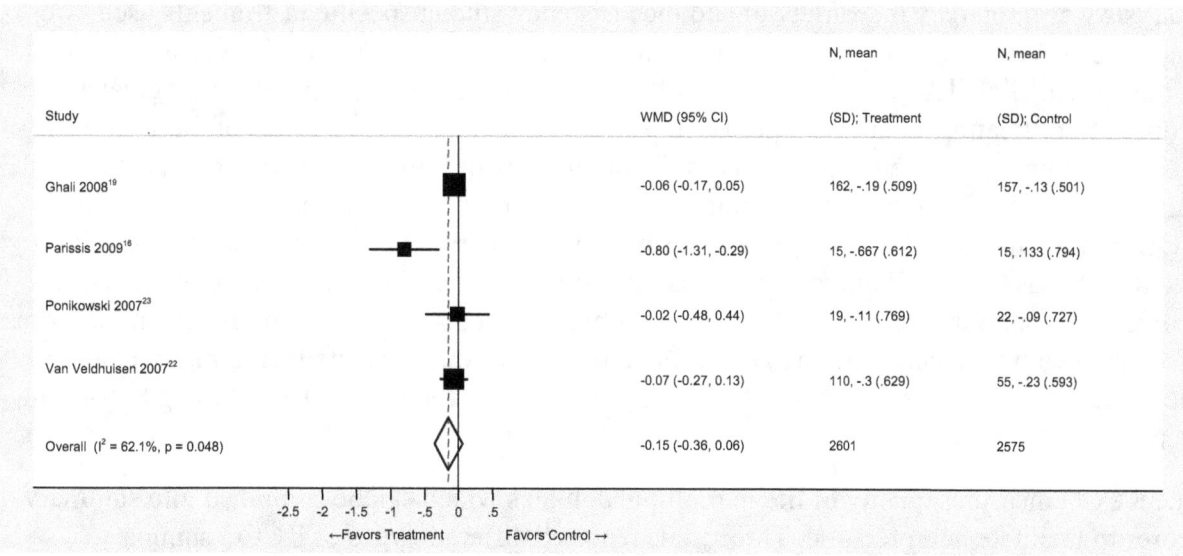

Six trials reported exercise distance or duration. Four of these trials reported the mean change in six-minute walk distance and found ESA use was associated with a marginally significant increase in distance walked, though results were quite different among the trials (mean change in meters walked: 74.4; 95% CI -0.16 to 149.0; I^2=88.7%) (Figure 5). Two trials reported change in exercise treadmill time using the Naughton protocol; the larger trial found no improvement associated with ESA use,[19] while a smaller trial found ESA use was associated with a small increase in exercise duration.[28] Exclusion of poorer quality studies did not alter results substantially, but such analyses are limited by the very small number of studies.

Figure 5. Change in six-minute walk distance (meters) in CHF patients: mean difference comparing ESA to control group

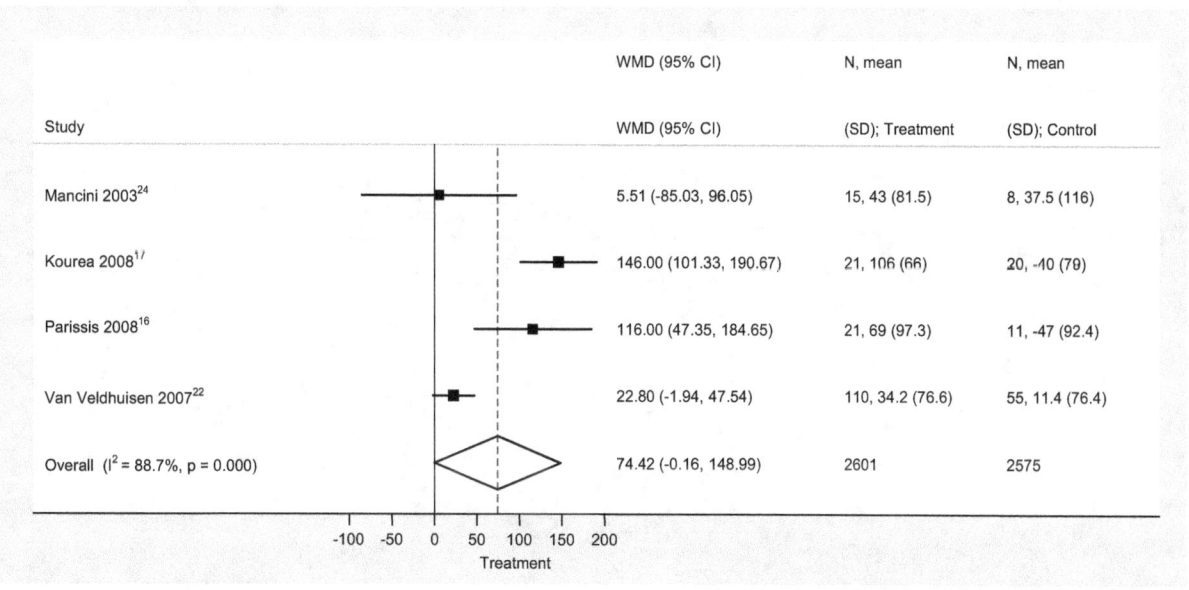

Quality of Life

Five trials reported quality of life measures as a primary or secondary outcome,[17, 19, 22-24] but analysis was limited by the variety of and inconsistency among specific instruments used. Most trials used several different methods for evaluating quality of life. Four trials evaluated change in the Patient Global Assessment scale.[19, 22-24] In two of these studies, a significantly greater proportion of treatment patients reported improvement than controls, but one of these studies had several important methodologic flaws, including lack of blinding, that could bias these subjective results.[24] The other trial found no improvement in two simultaneously measured QOL instruments including the Minnesota Living with Heart Failure Questionnaire (MLHFQ) and the Kansas City Cardiomyopathy Questionnaire (KCCQ).[23] Four trials reported MLHFQ scores,[19, 22-24] but only one trial with high risk of bias showed a significant improvement in scores associated with treatment.[24] Kourea et al. found treatment was associated with improvement in the Duke Activity Status Index (DASI), Beck Depression Inventory (BDI) and Zung Self-rating Depression Scale (SDS).[17]

The KCCQ measures quality of life in multiple domains which can be combined into summary scores to facilitate interpretation. Three trials reported different types of KCCQ summary scores without defining which domains were used in each summation.[17, 22, 23] One trial reported a significant difference between groups in mean change from baseline of a KCCQ "total symptom score": 8.2 v 1.5, p=0.027.[22] Another trial noted significant improvements in a KCCQ "functional score" (21 +/- 19 v 2 +/- 11, p=0.004), as well as a KCCQ "summary" score (20 +/- 20 v 6 +/- 14, p=0.04).[17]

Mortality

Nine trials reporting at least one death in the treatment or control group found ESA use was associated with a marginally significant increased mortality risk (RR 1.11; 95% CI 0.99 – 1.24; I^2=0.0%). An analysis of the six trials with low risk of bias found very similar results (Figure 6).

These findings are largely driven by two large trials with extended follow-up and very high event rates. Indeed, a sensitivity analysis without these two trials showed ESAs had a neutral effect on mortality (RR 0.79, 95% CI 0.51 – 1.22; I^2=0.0%). One of the trials compared aggressive (goal hematocrit 42%) to less aggressive (goal hematocrit 30%) epoietin titration in patients with end-stage renal disease and heart failure and/or ischemic heart disease.[26] After a prolonged follow-up of 29 months, the authors found a 20 percent increase in the risk of all-cause mortality, and most of the events were of cardiovascular origin. Another large trial compared darbepoietin to placebo in patients with type 2 diabetes and chronic kidney disease. A prespecified analysis of the large subgroup with comorbid heart disease showed a non-significant increased risk of death in the treatment group after a similarly long follow-up period.[14, 29]

Figure 6. All-cause mortality in patients with CHF or CHD – studies with low risk of bias: ESA vs. control

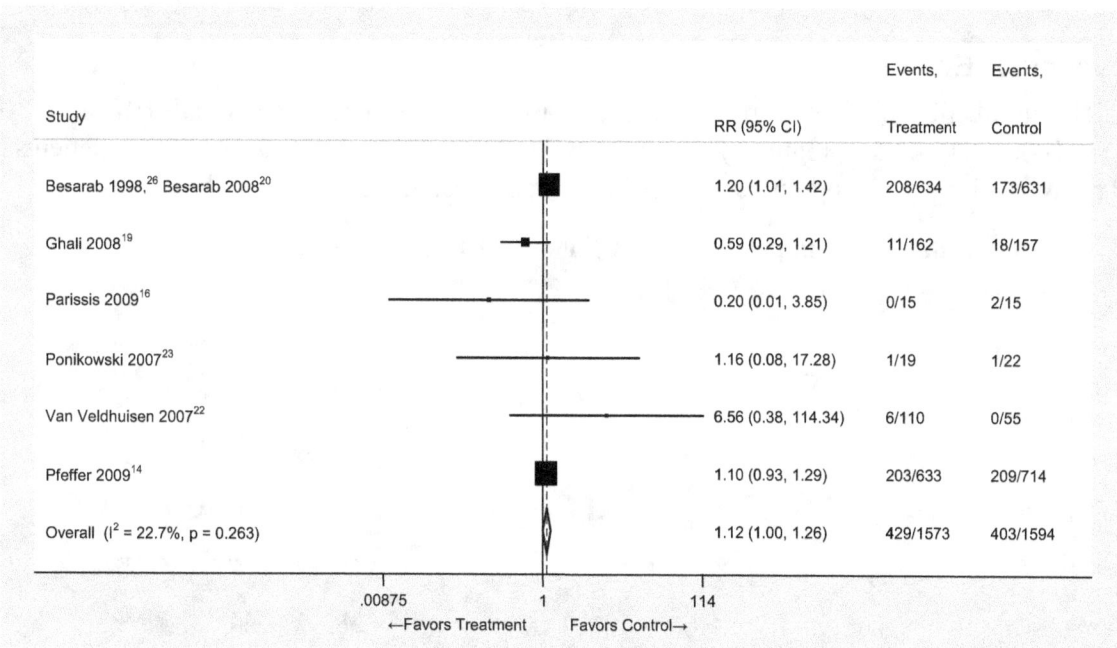

Hospitalizations

Six trials found ESA treatment was associated with a reduction in hospitalizations (RR 0.70, 95% CI 0.57 – 0.87; $I^2=37.7\%$), but, again, this benefit largely disappeared when we included only the higher quality trials (Figure 7).

Figure 7. Risk of one or more hospitalizations in patients with CHF or CHD – studies with low risk of bias: ESA vs. Control

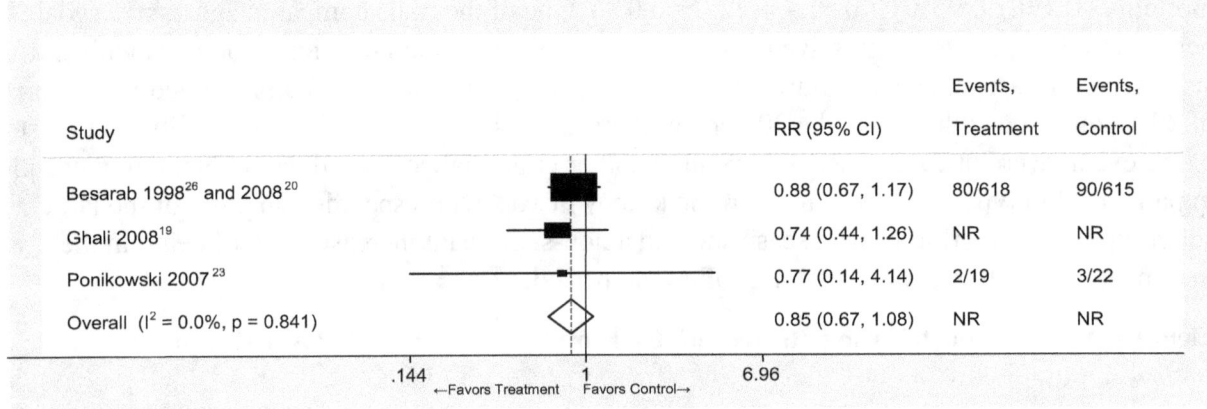

Cardiovascular Events

ESAs had a neutral effect on the occurrence of cardiovascular events across seven trials (RR 0.96, 95% CI 0.85 – 1.08; $I^2=41.5\%$, Figure 8). The only trial showing a benefit focused on CHD patients, and had many significant methodologic weaknesses which threaten the validity of the results.[27]

Figure 8. Cardiovascular events in patients with CHF or CHD: ESA vs. control

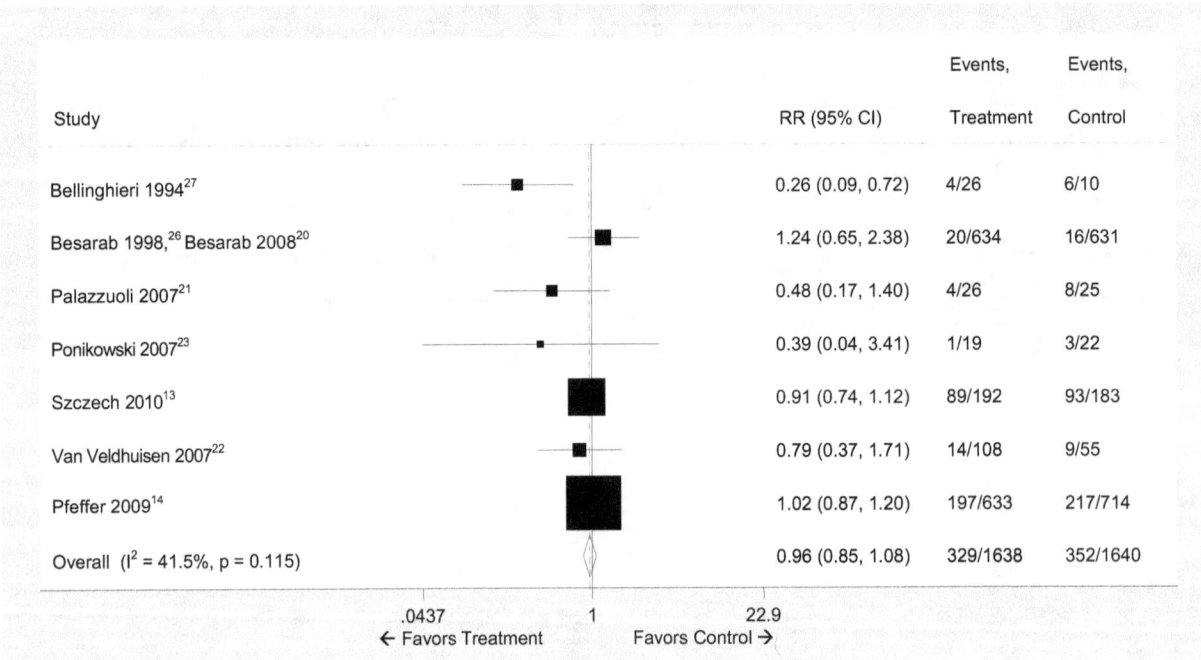

Cerebrovascular Events

There were very few cerebrovascular events among the four trials reporting this outcome (Figure 9). There was an increased risk of stroke associated with ESA use in the TREAT trial among patients with diabetes and chronic kidney disease (RR 1.92, 95% CI 1.38 – 2.68),[30] but these data are not reported separately for the large subgroup of heart disease patients.

Figure 9. Cerebrovascular events in patients with CHF or CHD: ESA vs. control

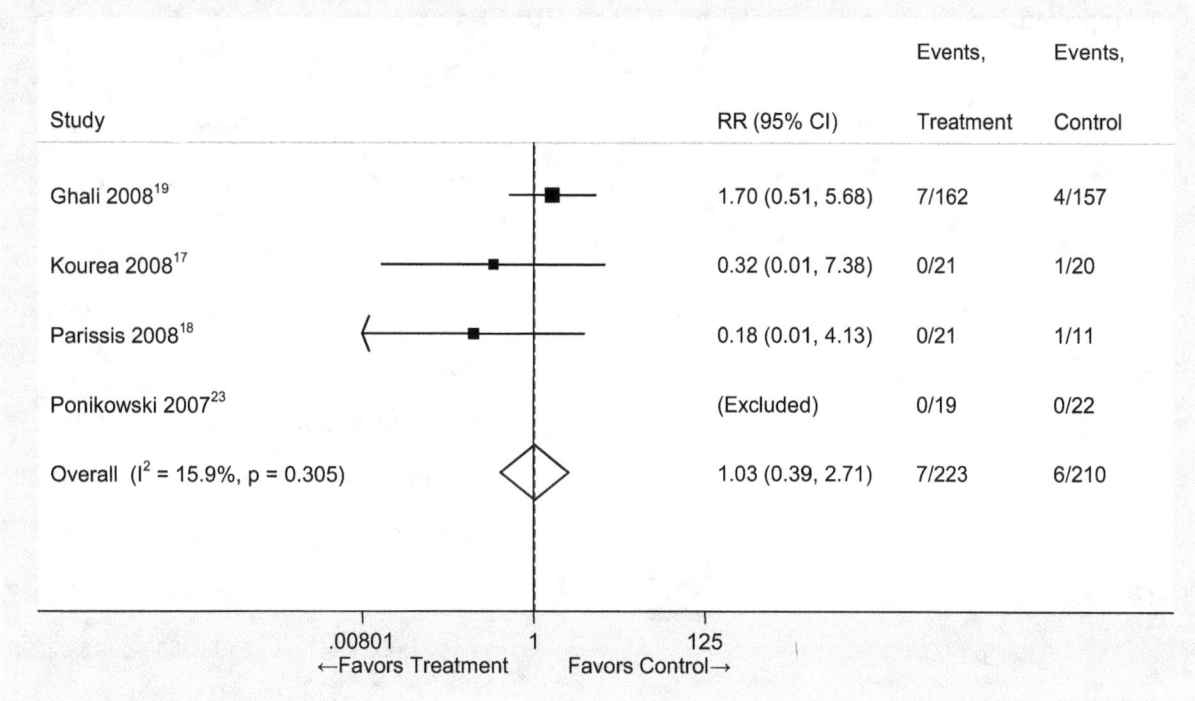

Study	RR (95% CI)	Events, Treatment	Events, Control
Ghali 2008[19]	1.70 (0.51, 5.68)	7/162	4/157
Kourea 2008[17]	0.32 (0.01, 7.38)	0/21	1/20
Parissis 2008[18]	0.18 (0.01, 4.13)	0/21	1/11
Ponikowski 2007[23]	(Excluded)	0/19	0/22
Overall (I^2 = 15.9%, p = 0.305)	1.03 (0.39, 2.71)	7/223	6/210

.00801   1   125
←Favors Treatment   Favors Control→

Other Harms

Combined results from seven trials suggest ESA use may be associated with excess risk of hypertension (RR 1.11, 95% CI 1.00 – 1.24; I^2= 0.0%), though the findings are again dominated by one large trial.[14] The finding of excess risk became non-significant when we excluded this trial (RR 1.25, 95 % CI 0.65 – 2.38; I^2=0.0%). Reported hypertension events in the other trials were rare, but the quality of adverse event reporting was unclear and the definitions used varied widely (Figure 10).

Figure 10. Hypertension events in patients with CHF or CHD: ESA vs. control

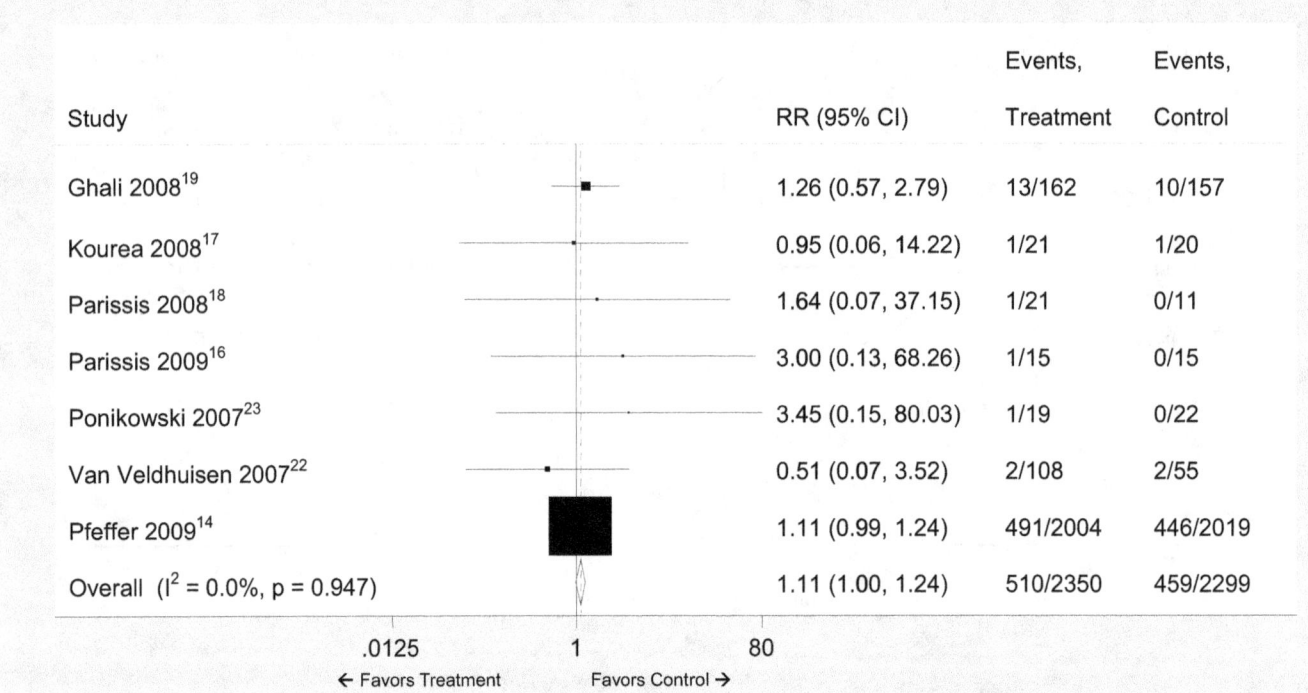

Study	RR (95% CI)	Events, Treatment	Events, Control
Ghali 2008[19]	1.26 (0.57, 2.79)	13/162	10/157
Kourea 2008[17]	0.95 (0.06, 14.22)	1/21	1/20
Parissis 2008[18]	1.64 (0.07, 37.15)	1/21	0/11
Parissis 2009[16]	3.00 (0.13, 68.26)	1/15	0/15
Ponikowski 2007[23]	3.45 (0.15, 80.03)	1/19	0/22
Van Veldhuisen 2007[22]	0.51 (0.07, 3.52)	2/108	2/55
Pfeffer 2009[14]	1.11 (0.99, 1.24)	491/2004	446/2019
Overall (I^2 = 0.0%, p = 0.947)	1.11 (1.00, 1.24)	510/2350	459/2299

.0125   1   80

← Favors Treatment   Favors Control →

One large trial in end-stage renal disease patients found an increase in the risk of thrombosis – mainly of vascular access sites – associated with aggressive epoietin titration (RR 1.37, 95% CI 1.17 – 1.61).[26] The risk of venous thromboembolism was similarly increased in another trial of patients with chronic kidney disease and diabetes (RR 1.80, 95% CI 1.08 – 2.98), though data for the cardiac disease subgroup were not reported separately.[14] On the other hand, only two other studies reported the occurrence of venous thromboembolic events with no difference seen between groups.[19, 22]

Hemoglobin Target

We were not able to determine how anemia severity and hemoglobin change influenced outcomes in the placebo-controlled trials. Almost all the small trials comparing ESAs to placebo in heart failure patients included patients with moderate anemia and a mean baseline hemoglobin within the narrow 10 – 12 g/dL range. In all cases, ESA use was associated with a significant increase in hemoglobin (mean increase range 1.6 – 2.8 g/dL). In order to better understand the influence of baseline hemoglobin and change in hemoglobin on outcomes, we conducted the two following sensitivity analyses for all outcomes and found no substantive difference in results:

1) exclusion of studies in which the mean baseline hemoglobin < 11 g/dL; and 2) exclusion of studies in which the mean increase in hemoglobin associated with ESA use was < 2 g/dL. However, the utility of such subgroup analysis is limited by the relatively small number of trials, and also by concurrent characteristics which could influence results. For instance, exclusion of studies with mean baseline hemoglobin < 11 g/dL examining change in NYHA scores left only the poorer quality studies. Furthermore, there may not have been enough variation in mean baseline hemoglobin and change in hemoglobin across studies given the relatively small sample of trials.

The best evidence evaluating the influence of hemoglobin targets comes from the three trials (or subgroups of trials) of patients with comorbid chronic kidney and heart disease, in which ESAs titrated to normal or near-normal targets were compared to ESAs titrated to lower targets (hemoglobin 9 – 11.3 g/dL).[13, 14, 20] None of the trials found a benefit from aggressive ESA use and, in fact, two of the trials found a significant increase in venous thromboembolic risk and a near-significant increase in mortality.[14, 20]

No trials in heart disease patients have evaluated the effects of more moderate hemoglobin targets (e.g. hemoglobin 10 – 12 g/dL) compared to lower targets.

In Progress Trials

Two trials of ESAs in heart failure are ongoing. The Reduction of Events with Darbepoetin alfa in Heart Failure (RED-HF) study is an international, multicenter, randomized and placebo-controlled trial.[31] The intent is to recruit ~2600 optimally treated patients with low ejection fraction (~40%) and symptomatic CHF with a Hgb concentration 9.0 – 12.0 g/dL. Patients will be administered darbepoetin every two weeks, titrated to a goal Hgb of >= 13.0 g/dL, with oral iron repletion as needed. The primary outcome is time to death from any cause or first hospital admission for worsening CHF. The secondary outcomes include mean change in KCCQ scores at six months. Started in June 2006, this event-driven, industry-sponsored trial is estimated to finish in 2014.

Also expected are results from the Anemia in Heart Failure With a Preserved Ejection Fraction trial.[32] This randomized, placebo-controlled trial is examining the effects of weekly erythropoietin, also titrated to a target hemoglobin of 13 g/dL, in 80 patients with anemia and heart failure and a preserved ejection fraction. They will evaluate the primary outcomes of left ventricular end diastolic volume at six months, as well as secondary outcomes of peak oxygen consumption, six-minute walk duration, KCCQ scores, hospitalization, and others. Started in July 2007, it is anticipated to be completed by March 2012.

KEY QUESTION #2. In patients with CHF or CHD, what are the health outcome benefits and harms of using iron to treat iron deficiency with or without anemia?

Summary

Two small and one large, well-conducted multicenter trials show that IV iron can improve short-term exercise tolerance and quality of life in patients with symptomatic systolic heart failure and iron deficiency, with or without anemia. The impact on distal health outcomes such as mortality and cardiovascular events remains undertested, as do the long-term effects of such treatment. The evidence supporting symptomatic benefit most closely applies to patients with NYHA III heart failure and evidence of low iron stores.

Details

We included three trials of IV iron in patients with iron deficiency. Results are largely dominated by one recent trial that studied the effect of iron infusion on patients with iron deficiency with or without anemia.[33]

The FAIR-HF (Ferinject Assessment in Patients with Iron Deficiency and Chronic Heart Failure) trial is a randomized, double-blind, multicenter trial that evaluated the efficacy of intravenous-iron infusion on symptoms and submaximal exercise capacity in a cohort of patients with chronic mild or moderate heart failure due to left ventricular systolic dysfunction. The study enrolled 459 stable outpatients with NYHA class II or III heart failure, low ejection fraction, and iron deficiency as defined by a ferritin < 100 µg/dL or between 100 – 299 µg/dL if the transferrin saturation was < 20 percent. Pre-specified primary endpoints included self-reported Patient Global Assessment and NYHA functional class after 24 weeks of therapy. Secondary endpoints included distance walked in six minutes and health-related quality of life. Patients receiving IV iron received 200 mg infusion of ferric carboxymaltose with repeat dosing until iron repletion was achieved (correction phase) and then every four weeks during the maintenance phase, which started at week eight or week twelve, depending on the required iron-repletion dose. Control patients received an IV saline placebo with the same dosing schedule.

Patient characteristics, which were well-matched between the two groups at baseline, are detailed in Table 2. Most patients had NYHA Class III symptoms and moderate to severe systolic dysfunction. Only half the patients were anemic (HHgb ≤ 12g/dL), but most had ferritin levels < 100.

Patients in the treatment group were more likely to report they were much or moderately improved on the Patient Global Assessment compared with control patients (50 v 28%, OR 2.51; 95% CI 1.75 – 3.61). Iron treated patients also showed improvement in NYHA functional class (OR for improvement by one class, 2.40; 95% CI 1.55 – 3.71). Improvements in Patient Global Assessment and NYHA scores were observed in both prespecified subgroups of patients with and without anemia (Hgb ≤ 12g/dL). Significant improvements were also seen in secondary endpoints, including an increased distance on the six-minute walk test (313 meters compared with 277 meters) and quality of life assessments (EQ5-D, where higher score is better, of 63 vs. 57).

The FAIR-HF trial was large and well-conducted, but there are several limitations of note. It relied on subjective primary endpoints, though the strong study design should minimize the risk of biased results. The size of the study and relatively short follow-up period limit its ability to examine intervention effects on more distal health outcomes such as mortality. Finally, there were too few patients with NYHA class II heart failure to meaningfully apply results to this group of patients.

We also included two smaller trials of iron therapy. The first randomized 40 patients with iron deficiency, anemia, chronic heart failure and chronic kidney disease to receive 200 mg of intravenous iron sucrose or saline weekly for five weeks.[34] Investigators found that after six months, participants who received iron sucrose had significant improvement in MLHFQ score, decreased levels of N-terminal pro-brain natriuretic peptide (117.5 +/- 87.4 pg/ml vs. 450.9 +/-248.8 pg/ml, $p<0.01$) and C-reactive protein (2.3 +/- 0.8 mg/l vs. 6.5 +/-3.7 mg/l, $p <0.01$), an increase in left ventricular ejection fraction percentage (35.7 +/- 4.7 vs. 28.8 +/- 2.4), and distance on the six-minute walk test.

The FERRIC-HF (Ferric Iron Sucrose in Heart Failure) trial randomized 35 patients and measured the effect of 200 mg of intravenous iron sucrose compared with placebo on exercise tolerance and QOL.[35] The lack of blinding contributes to a high risk of bias given the subjective nature of the functional status and QOL outcomes. Also, substantially more patients in the intervention group dropped out of the study (16 v 9%).

Table 2. Characteristics of randomized controlled trials of iron therapy in patients with CHF or CHD

Study setting and design	Characteristics of patient population, T v C	Results, N(%), T v C	Quality assessment
Anker, 2009[33] FAIR-HF Multicenter randomized controlled trial, international 24 weeks Ferric carboxymaltose IV 200 mg weekly until repleted, then q 4 weeks v saline 4 mL	N: 304 v 155 % male: 47.6 v 45.2 % white: 99.7 v 100 Mean age: 67.8 v 67.4 Mean LEVF%: 31.9 v 33.0 % NYHA II: 17.4 v 18.7 % NYHA III: 82.6 v 81.3 % RAAS blockers: 92.4 v 91.0 Baseline GFR: 63.8 v 64.8 Baseline ferritin: 52.5 v 60.1 Baseline TSAT%: 17.7 v 16.7 Baseline Hgb: 11.9 v 11.9	Mean change in HHgb: 1.1 v 0.6 Mortality: 5 (3.4) v 4 (5.5) Cardiac events: 46 events in 38 pts (27.6%) v 49 events in 33 pts (50.2%), p=0.01 First cardiovascular hospitalization: HR 0.53 (95% CI 0.25-1.09, p 0.08) Functional status/activity tolerance: NYHA, OR for improvement by 1 class: 2.40 (95% CI 1.55-3.71) Patient global assessment, OR for improvement: 2.51 (95% CI 1.75-3.61) 6 minute walk (meters): 313 v 277 Quality of life outcomes: Kansas City Cardiomyopathy Questionnaire Score: 66 v 59 EQ-5D Score: 63 v 57 Adverse events: GI event: 29 events in 24 pts (16.9%) v 7 events in 5 pts (6.9%), p=0.06 Respiratory event: 9 events in 9 pts (6.2%) v 13 events in 10 pts (14.2%), p=0.06	Overall: low risk of bias Funding source: Vifor Pharma
Okonko 2008[35] Randomized controlled trial 2 centers in Europe 18 weeks Iron sucrose IV in varied doses (according to a formula in paper) weekly for four weeks then q 4 weeks for four months; no control	N: 24 v 11 % male: 71 v 73 % white: 88 v 91 Mean age: 64 v 62 % CAD: 79 v 73 LVEF%: 30 v 29 RAAS blockers: 96 v 91 Baseline Cr: 1.23 v 1.17 (mg/dL) Baseline ferritin: 62 v 88 Baseline TSAT%: 20 v 21 Baseline Hgb: 12.6 v 12.2	Mean change in Hgb: 0.5 v 0.4 Mortality: 1/24 (4.2%) v 0 Hospitalizations: 3/24 (12%) v 3/11 (27%) Functional status/activity tolerance: NYHA: 2.1 v 2.6 Mean change NYHA -0.4 v 0.2, p = 0.007 Mean change exercise duration (s): 45 v -15 Patient global assessment: 1.5 v -0.2, p = 0.002 Mean change MLHFQ: -10 v 3, p = 0.07 Adverse events: abdominal pain -2/24 (8%) v 0 TIA - 1/24 (4%) v 0	Overall: unclear risk of bias Funding source: Vifor International
Toblli, 2007[34] Randomized controlled trial 6 months Iron sucrose IV 200 mg v saline 200 ml weekly x 5 weeks.	N: 20 v 20 % male: NR % white: NR Mean age: 76 v 74 % CAD: 60 v 55 Mean LVEF%: 31.3 v 30.8 % RAAS blockers: 95 v 100 Baseline GFR: 39.8 v 37.7 Baseline ferritin: 73.0 v 70.6 Baseline TSAT%: 20 v 20 Baseline Hgb: 10.3 v 10.2	Mean change in Hgb: +1.5 v -0.4 Mean change in CrCl: +5.1 v -6.0, p<0.01Hospitalizations: 0/20 v 5/20 (20%), p<0.01 Functional status/activity tolerance: MLHFQ score: 41 v 59, p<0.01 Mean change in MLHFQ score: -19 v -6 6 minute walk (meters): 240.1 v 184.5 , p<0.01	Overall: low risk of bias.

KEY QUESTION #3. In patients with CHF or CHD, what are the health outcome benefits and harms of treating anemia with red blood cell transfusions?

Summary

We found 35 studies that examine the association between red blood cell transfusion and clinical outcomes in patients with CHD or CHF. Ten of these studies evaluated transfusion use in the perioperative period; the remaining reports, all but one published since 2001, focused on the non-surgical population. Three of these studies were subgroup analyses of the same registry;[36-38] thus, in the end, we found 23 unique studies of the potential benefits and harms of transfusion outside of the perioperative period in patients with ischemic heart disease and/or CHF.

Outside of the surgical setting, red blood cell transfusion has been evaluated as a treatment for anemia in heart disease in two controlled trials: one found no difference in survival from more aggressive transfusion above a threshold hemoglobin 10 g/dL,[39] while the other found a higher incidence of heart failure in patients transfused to that level, without a difference in survival.[40]

Twenty-one additional observational studies have been conducted in patients undergoing percutaneous coronary intervention (PCI) or admitted with acute coronary syndrome, myocardial infarction, or decompensated heart failure. Inconsistency of findings and methodological weaknesses complicate the interpretation of results, but several themes emerge: 1) the evidence strongly suggests that transfusion has no benefit and may be harmful in patients with heart disease and hemoglobin >10 g/dL, with the possible exception of those with ST-elevation myocardial infarction; 2) outcomes do not appear to improve with transfusion in non-ST-elevation ACS patients with hemoglobin levels down to the 8 – 9 g/dL range; 3) transfusion is consistently associated with higher mortality risk in the unselected PCI population, across multiple studies with mean nadir hemoglobin of 8 – 9 g/dL; and 4) the elevated risk in the PCI population is seen in patients with anemia related or unrelated to bleeding but may be higher in the non-bleeding anemic population. There is no evidence to guide decision-making in the stable coronary disease population, and the two studies in decompensated heart failure have conflicting results.

The literature evaluating the use of perioperative transfusion in patients with heart disease is concentrated primarily on the cardiac surgery population but does include several studies in vascular and orthopedic surgery and one in the general non-cardiac surgery population. Seven perioperative randomized controlled trials have been conducted, and each found no difference in survival or cardiovascular complications between patients transfused to a higher versus lower target hemoglobin. In the observational cohorts, transfusion did not appear to offer any protection; and in one study in the vascular surgery setting, mortality and myocardial infarction rates were higher overall in the transfused group, a harm in subgroup analysis limited to those transfused at a hemoglobin ≥ 9 g/dL.[41]

Non-operative Setting

Randomized Controlled Trials

Only 2 of the 23 studies in nonsurgical populations were randomized controlled trials (Table 3).[39, 40] The TRICC trial, published in 1999, remains the only large controlled trial of transfusion strategies in hospitalized patients.[42] This landmark study randomized 838 euvolemic, non-bleeding, critically ill patients with hemoglobin < 9 g/dL to one of two transfusion thresholds: hemoglobin of 7 g/dL (restrictive transfusion strategy) or 10 g/dL (liberal strategy). They found no significant difference between the two groups in mortality in the hospital or at 30 days, or in other clinical outcomes including cardiac events, pulmonary or infectious complications, organ dysfunction scores, and length of stay. Importantly, the trend suggested the potential for higher mortality and more cardiac events in patients treated to the higher hemoglobin level. In the subgroups of patients younger than 55 years of age or with APACHE II scores of 20 or lower, the mortality rate was statistically significantly higher in the liberally transfused group.

In 2001, the TRICC authors published a post-hoc subgroup analysis focusing on patients with cardiovascular disease in general and ischemic heart disease in particular.[39] Once again, there were no significant differences in any clinical outcome. However, the trend toward improved survival with a restrictive transfusion strategy disappeared in the general cardiovascular disease population, and in the ischemic heart disease subgroup, there was a higher mortality rate in the restrictive group, though the difference was nonsignificant (30 day mortality 21.1% versus 26.1% with liberal and restrictive strategies, respectively; p=0.38). Like the TRICC trial population overall, the ischemic heart disease subgroup was severely ill with multiple comorbidities (mean APACHE II scores of 23, 87% requiring mechanical ventilation).

Cooper et al. performed a pilot trial (CRIT) designed to evaluate conservative versus liberal transfusion strategies specifically in patients with acute myocardial infarction.[40] They randomized 45 patients with hematocrit under 30 percent to a transfusion trigger of 24 percent (conservative strategy), with a target hematocrit 24 – 27 percent, or a trigger of 30 percent (liberal strategy), with a target of 30 – 33 percent. They found a higher rate of the primary endpoint, a composite of in-hospital death, recurrent MI, or new/worsening heart failure, in the liberally transfused group compared to the conservative group (38% versus 13%; p=0.046). The difference was explained entirely by a higher incidence of new or worsening CHF.

An additional study, the Myocardial Ischemia and Transfusion trial, began two years ago and is now collecting final outcomes data.[43] This multicenter, randomized, controlled trial aimed to enroll 200 anemic patients hospitalized with acute coronary syndrome, including both STEMI and NSTE-ACS, or stable CAD undergoing cardiac catheterization during the index hospitalization. Like the TRICC and CRIT trials, patients were assigned to a restrictive (< 8 g/dL) or liberal (< 10 g/dL) transfusion threshold and were observed for clinical outcomes including mortality, myocardial ischemia, stroke, heart failure, infectious complications, and readmission.

Observational Studies

Given the sparse and the inconsistent data from the trial literature, clinical decision-making appears largely guided by an imperfect body of evidence characterized by conflicting observational data. We reviewed these observational studies, in part to clarify their utility in guiding transfusion treatment decisions (Table 4).

Because of the observational nature of these studies, the decision to transfuse patients was based on clinical judgment which, in turn, would be naturally influenced by severity of illness, symptoms, and observation of bleeding. All the included observational studies suffer from the possibility of residual confounding and are all, therefore, of lower quality than the evidence provided by randomized controlled trials. However, there were methodologic differences amongst observational studies. For instance, some accounted for bleeding and conducted propensity to transfuse adjustments, while others did not. These factors are summarized in Appendix C, Table 3.

Percutaneous Coronary Intervention

Nine observational studies looked exclusively at populations undergoing percutaneous coronary intervention; six included all indications,[36-38, 44-48] and three examined PCI solely in the setting of acute MI.[49-51]

In those studies that recorded it, 1.8 – 6.7 percent of unselected patients undergoing PCI received PRBC transfusion; rates were higher in those studies for which anemia was an inclusion criterion. A substantial proportion of patients who received transfusions did so because of major bleeding (22 – 100%), and median nadir hematocrit prior to transfusion ranged across studies from 24 to 30 percent. After adjustment for potential confounding factors in multivariable analyses, transfusion was associated with worse survival in all studies but one;[36-38] it found no significant relationship between transfusion exposure and death or MI, both in cohorts with hematocrit < 27 percent and 24 – 30 percent. The association between transfusion and increased mortality appeared stronger in non-bleeding patients,[44, 51] but was also noted in several studies that examined patients with major bleeding.[44-46]

Acute Coronary Syndrome/Myocardial Infarction

Twelve observational studies evaluated transfusion in the setting of acute coronary syndrome or myocardial infarction; four included only patients with non-ST-elevation ACS,[52-55] two included patients exclusively with ST-elevation MI,[50, 56] and six examined mixed ST/non-ST elevation ACS populations. Of these, three included predominately STEMI patients,[51, 57, 58] two had a majority NSTE-ACS population,[59, 60] and one did not record the breakdown.[49] PCI rates ranged from 10 to 100 percent and transfusion rates from 4 to 30 percent across cohorts. Nadir hematocrit among patients who were transfused averaged from 25 to 29 percent in those studies that recorded it.

Eight of the ACS/AMI studies did find an association between transfusion and higher risk of death, including the three studies that focused exclusively on AMI patients undergoing PCI;[49-51] three involving patients with high-risk non-ST-elevation ACS,[52-54] and two examining patients primarily with ST-elevation myocardial infarction.[56, 58] One additional study found no relationship between transfusion status and in-hospital mortality in a mixed ST/non-ST-elevation ACS population, regardless of whether the transfusion was bleeding-related or for non-specific anemia.[60]

Six studies examined whether mortality risk varies according to hemoglobin level, but they had varied results and used different thresholds for their stratified analyses, making it difficult to draw firm conclusions.[52, 54, 55, 57-59]

Wu et al. examined a cohort of nearly 79,000 Medicare beneficiaries 65 years of age or older who were hospitalized with confirmed acute MI and were not actively bleeding.[59] They found a consistent association between transfusion and improved survival in patients with hematocrit values on admission of 30 percent or less, stronger in each successively lower hematocrit category. This benefit was lost in patients with hematocrit above 33 percent, and risk of death at 30 days was statistically significantly higher with transfusion once hematocrit rose above 36 percent.

Meanwhile, Rao et al. analyzed 24,112 patients who had been enrolled in three large international ACS trials (GUSTO IIB, PURSUIT, PARAGON B).[52] They found that receipt of transfusion predicted increased risk of death and death/MI at 30 days. After stratifying results by nadir hematocrit, they noted no association between transfusion exposure and mortality with a hematocrit of 25 percent or below, but they found a highly increased probability of death at 30 days with transfusion at a nadir hematocrit of 30 percent or higher.

Sabatine et al. performed a post-hoc meta-analysis of 16 prior TIMI cardiac trials, finding that transfusion appeared to confer a protective effect in terms of cardiovascular mortality in patients with STEMI and admission hemoglobin less than 12 g/dL.[57] Meanwhile, there was a non-significant trend towards worse outcomes in STEMI with transfusion at hemoglobin level greater than 12 g/dL; and in the NSTE-ACS population, they noted an association between transfusion and higher risk for a combined mortality and cardiovascular event endpoint at all hemoglobin levels.

Of the three remaining studies that performed stratified analyses, transfusion was found to be of potential benefit in acute MI patients with nadir hemoglobin 8 g/dL or less,[58] and nonsignificant trends toward improved outcomes were noted in NSTE-ACS patients with hemoglobin at presentation less than 9 g/dL,[54] and NSTE-ACS patients with hematocrit 24 percent or less.[55] In each case, transfusion at hemoglobin or hematocrit levels higher than these thresholds was associated with increased mortality.

Heart Failure

Two observational studies evaluated patients with acute decompensated heart failure,[61, 62] with conflicting results. Garty et al. evaluated 2,335 patients admitted for acute decompensated heart failure to public hospitals in Israel.[61] They found that transfusion appeared to confer lower risk of death at 30 days, with trends toward benefit in-hospital, at one year and at four years. Meanwhile, Kao et al. noted higher adjusted in-hospital mortality with transfusion in a large cohort of patients hospitalized for heart failure in California.[62] This association was noted in both anemic and non-anemic patients but was much stronger in the non-anemic cohort.

Perioperative Setting

Cardiac Surgery

There were four randomized controlled trials of which two enrolled fewer than 40 patients total and were designed to evaluate primarily hemodynamic and lab parameters, while two were larger, enrolling 400 to 500 patients with primary clinical endpoints (Table 3). All were consistent in finding no difference in survival or cardiovascular complications with a conservative compared to a liberal transfusion strategy.[63-66]

Non-cardiac Surgery

Six studies, including three controlled trials and three observational studies, have reported outcomes based on transfusion status in patients with heart disease undergoing non-cardiac surgery. In the three controlled trials, performed in hip fracture and vascular surgery populations, there was no apparent benefit or harm from a more versus less aggressive transfusion strategy (Table 3).[67-69] By far, the largest of these studies, the FOCUS trial that enrolled over 2,000 patients undergoing hip fracture surgery, has only reported results in abstract form, with full publication expected in the very near future. The authors report no difference in mortality and functional status outcomes between the liberal and conservative transfusion groups. In the observational cohorts, transfusion did not appear to offer any protection, and in one study in the vascular surgery setting, mortality and myocardial infarction rates were higher overall in the transfused group, a harm in subgroup analysis limited to those transfused at a hemoglobin ≥ 9 g/dL (Table 3).[41, 68, 70]

Table 3. Randomized controlled trials of red blood cell transfusion for anemia in patients with CHD or CHF, stratified by patient setting

Study ID	Patient Population	N	Intervention		Transfusion Rate (%)		Rate of Major Bleeding (%)	Mean Achieved Hgb/Hct		Outcome	%		HR/OR adj or P value
			Liberal Hgb/Hct trigger	Restrictive Hgb/Hct trigger	Liberal	Restrictive		Liberal	Restrictive		Liberal	Restrictive	
Non-operative settings													
Cooper, 2011[40] CRIT trial	AMI (40% STEMI, 55.6% PCI) Hct ≤30% multicenter US, 2003-2009	45	Hct 30	Hct 24	100	54	0 (exclusion criterion)	Hct 30.6	Hct 27.9	mortality, in-hospital	5	8	p=1.0
										death/MI/CHF, in-hospital	38	13	p=0.046
										CHF, in-hospital	38	8	p=0.03
										mortality, 30 d	5	8	p=1.0
										death/MI/CHF, 30 d	60	20	p=0.02
Hebert, 2001[39] TRICC trial	ICU, 1° or 2° cardiovascular dx Hgb ≤9 g/dL post-hoc analysis, multicenter RCT Canada, 1994-1997	357 (44.8% restrictive)	Hgb 10	Hgb 7	100 (full study)	67 (full study)	0 (exclusion criterion)	Hgb 10.3	Hgb 8.5	mortality, 30 d	22.8	22.5	0.79 (0.45-1.43)
										mortality, 60 d	26.9	26.2	p=0.9
	Known ischemic heart disease only	257 (43.2% restrictive)								mortality, 30 d	21.1	26.1	p=0.38
										mortality, 60 d	24.5	28.8	p=0.48
Non-cardiac surgery													
Bush, 1997[67]	Vascular surgery (aortic/infrainguinal) (25% previous MI, 10% CHF) single center US, 1995-1996	99	Hgb 10	Hgb 9	NR	NR	NR	Hgb 11.0	Hgb 9.8	mortality, 30 d	8	8	p>0.6 for all
										MI, 30 d	4	2	
										cardiac events, 48 hrs	16	16	
Carson, 1998[68]	Hip fracture surgery (45.2% CV disease), Hgb <10 g/dL single center US, 1996-1997	84	Hgb 10	Hgb 8	100	45	NR	Hgb 10.7	Hgb 9.7	mortality, 60 d	4.8	11.9	NS
										death/immobility, 60 d	45.2	39.0	NS
Carson, 2009[69]	Hip fracture surgery CAD or risk factors (40% known CAD) post-op Hgb <10 g/dL multicenter N. America, 2003-2009	2016	Hgb 10	Hgb 8	100	NR	NR	Hgb 9.2	Hgb 7.9	mortality, 60 d	7.6	6.5	1.19 (0.76-1.86)
										death/immobility, 60 d	35	35	1.03 (0.85-1.23)
										readmissions			NS
										falls			NS
										fatigue			NS
Cardiac surgery													
Bracey, 1999[65]	Cardiac surgery single center US, 1997	428	Hgb 9	Hgb 8	64	60	NR	NR	NR	mortality, in-hospital	2.7	1.4	p=0.32
										MI, in-hospital	0.5	0	NS
Hajjar, 2010[66]	Cardiac surgery single center Brazil, 2009-2010	502	Hct 30	Hct 24	78	47	NR	Hct 31.8	Hct 28.4	mortality, 30 d	5	6	p=0.93
										death/shock/ARDS/dialysis, 30 d	10	11	p=0.85
										cardiac complications	21	24	p=0.27
Johnson, 1992[64]	Cardiac surgery single center US, dates NR	39	Hct 32	Hct 25	100	80	NR	Hct 31.3	Hct 28.4	mortality, in-hospital	0	0	NS
										MI/CVA/CHF, in-hospital	11.1	5	NS
Weisel, 1984[63]	Cardiac surgery single center Canada, dates NR	27	Hgb 12 (plus plasma for volume)	Hgb 7 (plus crystalloid for volume)	NR	NR	NR	Hgb 12.1	Hgb 8.9	mortality, 72 hrs	0	0	NS
										MI, 72 hrs	0	0	NS

Table 4. Observational studies of red blood cell transfusion for anemia in patients with CHD/CHF

Study ID	Patient Population	Design	Number	Transfusion Rate (%)	Rate of Major Bleeding (%)	Mean/Median Nadir Hct, Transfused Cohort (%)	Outcome	Crude % Transfused	Crude % Not Transfused	HR/OR adj
Percutaneous Coronary Intervention										
Chase, 2008[48]	PCI, all indications (64.9% ACS, STEMI rate NR) 4 centers in British Columbia, 1999-2005	Observational cohort, registry	38872	2.5	NR	NR	mortality, 30 d mortality, 1 yr	12.6 22.9	1.3 3.2	4.01 (3.08-5.22) 3.58 (2.94-4.36)
		Propensity score matched cohort	914	50			mortality, 30 d propensity matched mortality, 1 yr propensity matched	7.7 19.3	2 5.7	3.9 (1.89-8.0) 3.38 (2.22-5.14)
Doyle, 2008[47]	PCI, all indications (65.4% urgent/emergent; STEMI rate NR) Mayo Clinic, 1994-2005	Observational cohort, administrative database	17901	6.7	4.8 (overall) 38 (transfused cohort)	NR	mortality, 30 d 1-2 units ≥3 units mortality, 1 yr	24.6	13	8.9 (6.3-12.6) 18.1 (13.7-24.0) 2.02 (1.47-2.79)
Jani, 2007[49]	PCI, MI within prior 7 d (STEMI rate NR) anemia pre-PCI multicenter Michigan (BCBS),1997-2004	Observational cohort, registry	4623	22.3	NR	Hgb 10.0 (overall)	mortality, in-hospital MACE, in-hospital stroke/TIA	14.52 20.81 2.42	3.01 5.13 0.84	2.02 (1.47-2.79)
		Propensity score matched cohort	1196			transfused cohort NR but 87.8% Hgb <10	mortality, in-hospital, propensity matched stroke/TIA, propensity matched	12.71 2.01	7.36 2.01	
Jolicoeur, 2009[50]	PCI, STEMI multicenter multinational, 2004-2006	Observational cohort, post-hoc analysis of APEX-AMI trial	5532	3.9	81.7 (transfused cohort)	Hgb 8.7	mortality, 90 d CV death, 90 d MI, 90 d CHF, 90 d CVA, 90 d	26 16.7 7.8 15.2 4.9	4.1 3.5 2.6 4.4 1	2.16 (1.20-3.88)
Kim, 2007[45]	PCI, all indications (ACS/STEMI rates NR) Hct drop >10% single institution 2000-2002	Observational case-control, registry	146 txfused pts, 292 controls	NR	100	24	mortality, in hospital mortality, 1 yr	11 26	3.1 10.3	p=0.0008 2.42 (1.32-4.46)
Kinnaird, 2003[44]	PCI, all indications (2.4% AMI, 67.2% unstable angina) single center US, 1991-2000	Observational cohort, registry	10974	5.4	5.4 (overall) 41.8 (transfused cohort)	24.7	mortality, in-hospital major bleeding no bleeding mortality, 1 yr major bleeding no bleeding	9.2 10.6 10.3 28.4 22.7 36.8	0.6 5.1 0.4 5.4 13.6 5	2.0 (1.1-3.2) 1.9 (1.4-2.5)
Maluenda, 2009[38]	PCI, all indications (ACS/STEMI rates NR) Hct ≤ 27% post-PCI single US institution 2003-2007	Observational cohort, registry	379	53.5	NR	24.1	death/MI, 1 yr	26.6	17.2	1.1 (0.7-1.6)

Treatment of Anemia in Patients with Heart Disease: A Systematic Review

Study ID	Patient Population	Design	Number	Transfusion Rate (%)	Rate of Major Bleeding (%)	Mean/Median Nadir Hct, Transfused Cohort (%)	Outcome	Crude % Transfused	Crude % Not Transfused	HR/OR adj
Maluenda, 2009[36]	PCI, all indications (ACS/STEMI rates NR) Hct 24-30% post-PCI single US institution 2003-2007	Observational cohort, registry	625	30.2	9.6 (overall) 22.8 (transfused cohort)	26.5	death/MI, 30 d; mortality, 30 d; death/MI, 1 yr; mortality, 1 yr	15.8; 15.3; 28.6; 27.5	7.1; 6.9; 19.6; 18.5	1.4 (0.8-2.5); 1.4 (0.9-2.0)
	subgroup analysis, MI/shock		202				death/MI, 30 d; death/MI, 1 yr			1.3 (0.6-2.8); 0.9 (0.5-1.9)
	subgroup analysis, major bleeding		60		100 (transfused cohort)		death/MI, 30 d; death/MI, 1 yr	14; 27.9	11.8; 17.6	NS; NS
Maluenda, 2009[37]	PCI, all indications (ACS/STEMI rates NR) normal Hct pre-PCI w/ major bleeding single US institution 2003-2007	Observational cohort, registry	3738	1.6	100 (transfused cohort)	NR	death/MI, 1 yr	16.4	3.7	1.93 (0.81-4.17)
Nikolsky, 2009[51]	PCI, AMI (88% STEMI) multicenter multinational, 1997-1999	Observational cohort, post-hoc analysis of CADILLAC trial	2082	4	40.2 (transfused cohort)	29.9 (53.7% Hct >30)	mortality, 30 d; mortality, 1 yr; MACE, 1 yr	13.4; 23.9; 41	3.4; 16.6	4.71 (1.97-11.26); 3.16 (1.66-6.03)
	subgroup analysis, txfusion for major bleeding vs no bleed		33 major bleeding; 49 no bleed			28.5 (bleeding); ---; 30.4 (no evident bleeding)	mortality, 30 d; mortality, 1 yr; mortality, 30 d; mortality, 1 yr	6.1; 19; 18.4; 29.3		
Yatskar, 2007[46]	PCI, all indications (41.9% urgent/emergent; 24.0% AMI, STEMI rate NR) multicenter US, 1997-1999, 2001-2002	Observational cohort, registry	6656	1.8	1.8 (overall) 100 (transfused cohort)	NR	mortality, in-hospital; mortality, 1 yr	9.9; 18.8	1.2; 4.7	3.59 (1.66-7.77); 1.65 (1.01-2.70)

Acute Coronary Syndrome/Acute MI

Study ID	Patient Population	Design	Number	Transfusion Rate (%)	Rate of Major Bleeding (%)	Mean/Median Nadir Hct, Transfused Cohort (%)	Outcome	Crude % Transfused	Crude % Not Transfused	HR/OR adj
Aggarwal, 2011[60]	ACS (40% STEMI, 61% PCI) single center US, 2002-2006	Observational case-control	103 txfused pts, 185 controls	NA	42 (transfused cohort)	26.2	mortality, in-hospital; non-specific anemia; overt bleeding	19.4	10.8	1.8 (0.6-5.1); 0.9 (0.3-2.4); 2.7 (0.7-10.0)

Study ID	Patient Population	Design	Number	Transfusion Rate (%)	Rate of Major Bleeding (%)	Mean/Median Nadir Hct, Transfused Cohort (%)	Outcome	Crude % Transfused	Crude % Not Transfused	HR/OR adj
Alexander, 2008[55]	High-risk NSTE-ACS (61.2% PCI) multicenter US, 2004-2005	Observational cohort, registry (CRUSADE)	44242	10.4 (0.9%-79.2% lowest-highest quartile)	11.9 (overall; not given for transfused cohort)	25.7	mortality, in-hospital			
							Hct ≤ 24	11.8	15	0.67 (0.45-1.02)
							Hct 24.1-27	9.3	9.1	1.01 (0.79-1.30)
							Hct 27.1-30	7.3	6.1	1.18 (0.92-1.50)
							Hct >30	12.2	2.6	3.47 (2.30-5.23)
							death/MI, in-hospital			
							Hct ≤ 24	15.9	17.4	
							Hct 24.1-27	13.1	12.5	
							Hct 27.1-30	10.6	8.3	
							Hct >30	18.2	4	
							CHF, in-hospital			
							Hct ≤ 24	17.4	9.4	
							Hct 24.1-27	19.1	12.8	
							Hct 27.1-30	16.4	11.5	
							Hct >30	17.9	5.3	
Aronson, 2008[58]	AMI (81.8% STEMI; 27.8% PCI, 23.2% lytics) single Israeli institution, 2000-2006	Observational cohort, registry	2358	8.1	NR	Hgb 8.8	mortality, 6 mo, all	28.1	11.7	1.9 (p=0.001)
							Hgb ≤ 8			0.13 (CI 0.03-0.65)
							Hgb > 8			2.2 (CI 1.5-3.3)
							death/MI/CHF, 6 mo, all	41.1	19.6	1.4 (p=0.05)
							Hgb ≤ 8			0.24 (CI 0.07-0.75)
							Hgb > 8			1.6 (CI 1.1-2.2)
Rao, 2004[52]	NSTE-ACS (PCI rate NR) multicenter multinational, 1994-1999	Observational cohort, post-hoc meta-analysis of 3 RCTs (GUSTO IIB, PURSUIT, PARAGON B)	24112	10	NR (tracked bleeding and adjusted for but didn't report)	29	mortality, 30 d	8	3.1	3.94 (3.26-4.75)
							Hct 20			1.59 (0.95-2.66)
							Hct 25			1.13 (0.70-1.82)
							Hct 30			168.6 (7.5-3797.7)
							Hct 35			291.6 (10.3-8273.8)
							death/MI, 30 d	29.2	10	2.92 (2.55-3.35)
Sabatine, 2005[57]	ACS (63.7% STEMI, 34.8% revascularized), multicenter multinational, 1989-2001	Observational cohort, post-hoc meta-analysis of 13 TIMI trials	39922	3.9 (overall) 4.6 (STEMI) 2.7 (NSTE-ACS)	80 (transfused cohort)	NR	CV mortality, 30d, STEMI			
							Hgb < 12			0.42 (CI 0.20-0.89)
							Hgb ≥ 12			1.42 (CI0.94-2.17)
							MACE, 30 d, NSTE-ACS			1.54 (CI 1.14-2.09)
Shishehbor, 2009[56]	STEMI (18.5% PCI) multicenter multinational, 1994-1995	Observational cohort, post-hoc analysis of GUSTO IIB trial	3575	8.6	97 (transfused cohort) 0.6 (non-transfused)	25.1	mortality, 30 d	13.7	5.5	3.89 (2.66-5.68)
							MI, 30 d			3.44, p<0.001
							mortality, 6 mo	19.7	6.9	3.63 (2.67-4.95)
							MI, 6 mo			2.69, p<0.001
		Propensity score matched cohort	316				mortality, 1 yr	21.8	8.7	3.03 (2.25-4.08)
							mortality, 30 d, propensity matched			5.44 (3.21-9.22)
							mortality, 6 mo, propensity matched			4.81 (3.00-7.71)
							mortality, 1 yr, propensity matched			3.10 (2.18-4.40)

Treatment of Anemia in Patients with Heart Disease: A Systematic Review

Study ID	Patient Population	Design	Number	Transfusion Rate (%)	Rate of Major Bleeding (%)	Mean/Median Nadir Hct, Transfused Cohort (%)	Outcome	Crude % Trans-fused	Crude % Not Trans-fused	HR/OR adj
Singla, 2007[54]	Suspected NSTE-ACS (PCI rate NR) initial Hgb ≤11.5 g/dl single VA hospital, 2001-2005	Observational cohort, registry	370	29.7	NR	NR	mortality, 30 d death/MI, 30 d recurrent MI, 30 d	26.4 33.6 7.3	11.2 14.2 3.5	2.57 (1.41-4.69)
Wu, 2001[59]	AMI (28.3% STEMI, 24.9% cath, 10.3% PCI) all ≥65 yo multicenter US, 1994-1995	Observational cohort, administrative database	78974	4.7	0 (exclusion criterion)	NR	mortality, 30 d admission Hct 5-25 Hct 24.1-27 Hct 27.1-30 Hct 30.1-33 Hct 33.1-36 Hct 36.1-39 Hct >39			0.22 (0.11-0.45) 0.48 (0.34-0.69) 0.60 (0.47-0.76) 0.69 (0.53-0.89) 1.13 (0.89-1.44) 1.38 (1.05-1.80) 1.46 (1.18-1.81)
Yang, 2005[53]	High-risk NSTE-ACS (PCI rate NR) multicenter US, 2001-2004	Observational cohort, registry (CRUSADE)	85111 (overall), 74,271 non-CABG	14.9 (overall), 10.3 (non-CABG)	NR	26	mortality, in-hospital death/MI, in-hospital	11.5 13.4	3.8 5.8	1.67 (1.48-1.88) 1.44 (1.30-1.60)
Congestive Heart Failure										
Garty, 2009[61]	CHF, 1° admitting diagnosis multicenter Israel, 2003	Observational cohort, survey	2335	7.1	NR	Hgb 8.7	mortality, in-hospital mortality, 30 d mortality, 1 yr mortality, 4 yrs	10.8 11 39.6 69.5	5.2 8.5 28.5 59.5	0.48 (0.21-1.11) 0.29 (0.13-0.64) 0.74 (0.50-1.09) 0.86 (0.64-1.14)
		Propensity score matched cohort	206				mortality, in-hospital, propensity matched mortality, 30 d, propensity matched mortality, 1 yr, propensity matched mortality, 4 yrs propensity matched	8.7 9.7 38.8 72.8	14.6 18.4 42.7 76.7	
Kao, 2011[62]	CHF, 1° admitting diagnosis California hospitals, 2000-2006	Observational cohort, administrative database	596456	6.2	NR	NR; 27.1% had ICD-9 dx of anemia	mortality, in-hospital anemic non-anemic	8.37 7.09 17.46	3.96 4.43 3.81	3.8 (3.5-4.1) 1.7 (1.6-1.8)
Critical Illness										
Hebert, 1997[71]	ICU, 1° or 2° cardiovascular diagnosis, multicenter Canada, 1993	Observational cohort	1365	24.2	NR	Hgb 10.7	mortality, ICU Hgb < 9.5 Hgb < 9.5 + APACHE >20 + txfusion ≤6 units 1-3 units 4-6 units 7-10 units >10 units	28.8 31.2 34.3	17.5 27.4 55	0.61 (0.37-1.00) 0.49 (0.23-1.03) 0.96 (0.39-2.45) 0.64 (0.24-1.69)

38

Treatment of Anemia in Patients with Heart Disease: A Systematic Review

Study ID	Patient Population	Design	Number	Transfusion Rate (%)	Rate of Major Bleeding (%)	Mean/Median Nadir Hct, Transfused Cohort (%)	Outcome	Crude % Transfused	Crude % Not Transfused	HR/OR adj
Surgery										
Bursi, 2009[41]	Vascular surgery, major elective (hx CAD 26.7%, hx CHF 22.0%) single center Italy, date NR	Observational cohort	359	26.5	8.6	Hgb 9.2	mortality, 30 d	16.8	1.5	5.38 (1.45-20.0)
							Hgb 7-9			0.64 (0.13-3.18)
							Hgb ≥ 9			18.70 (3.12-112.1)
							MI, 30 d	21.1	6.8	2.23 (0.98-5.09)
							Hgb 7-9			3.07 (1.43-6.59)
							Hgb ≥ 9			0.83 (0.26-2.60)
							death/MI, 30 d	27.4	7.2	4.53 (1.69-12.12)
							mortality, 16.3 mo			4.02 (2.24-7.87)
							MI, 16.3 mo			2.02 (1.15-3.57)
							death/MI, 16.3 mo			2.67 (1.71-4.18)
Carson, 1998[68]	Hip fracture surgery, CV disease subgroup all ≥ 60 yo multicenter US, 1983-1993	Observational cohort	3783	42% (overall); NR for CV disease pts	NR		mortality, 30 d			1.07 (0.75-1.52)
							Hgb 7-7.9			NS
							Hgb 8-9.9			NS
							Hgb ≥ 10			NS
Glance, 2011[70]	Noncardiac surgery, non-emergent, cardiac disease, Hct <30%	Observational cohort, National Surgical Quality Improvement Program registry	10,100 (overall); cardiac disease subgroup NR	21.4 (overall)	NR	Baseline Hct 27.1	mortality, 30 d			NS

SUMMARY AND DISCUSSION

Anemia commonly complicates heart disease. Despite its association with poor outcomes and a biologically plausible argument supporting anemia correction, we found little evidence that use of ESAs or blood transfusions improve health outcomes in patients with heart disease. A limited evidence base consisting mainly of one trial suggests correction of iron deficiency in patients with symptomatic heart failure improves exercise tolerance and quality of life.

By far, the largest number of trials has examined ESAs in patients with heart failure, and most of these included patients with systolic heart failure. Though a grouped analysis of these mainly small, single-center studies shows some initial promise that ESAs may improve exercise tolerance, the evidence base is limited by inconsistent findings across trials, with some finding benefit and others finding no effect. There are a number of possible reasons for the discrepant results including differences in patient populations, treatment dosing and formulation, and outcomes examined. For example, the largest of the trials[19] enrolled slightly older patients and achieved a slightly smaller hemoglobin improvement with ESA use than did other trials finding a benefit. However, our analyses suggest that the clearest contributor to the discrepant findings was the quality of the individual studies themselves, with the poorer quality studies generally supporting a greater benefit from ESAs and the more rigorous trials finding a neutral effect.

Our review differs from a similar recent review of ESAs[72] for three main reasons: 1) we evaluated studies in both heart failure and CHD patients, though most studies focused on heart failure; 2) we conducted additional analyses investigating the impact of study quality on the overall results; and 3) we included studies of patients with advanced kidney disease if there were separately reported data for the subgroup of patients with comorbid heart disease. We felt the latter difference was justifiable because kidney disease is common among patients with heart disease, and we felt these data were important in understanding the potential benefits and harms in this population.

Though there were few excess harms reported in the smaller ESA trials of heart failure patients, the excess risk associated with ESAs in CKD populations[73] and cancer populations[74] is of concern. Moreover, our own analysis suggests the potential for serious harms associated with aggressive ESA use among the large proportion of patients with heart disease and comorbid CKD. On the other hand, these data may not apply to patients with symptomatic heart failure and reduced systolic function, and they do not elucidate the role of less aggressive ESA use, leaving us with very limited evidence with which to truly evaluate the balance of benefits and harms of ESAs in patients with heart disease. While the large RED-HF trial should more definitively establish the balance of benefits and harms of ESA use in patients with heart failure, the current uncertainty of benefit and the possibility of significant harms suggest widespread use of ESAs in patients with heart disease may be premature. For patients with comorbid chronic kidney disease, the recent cautious FDA recommendations seem reasonable, as they acknowledge the uncertainty of the role of ESA use and suggest that, if they are to be used at all, patients should have Hgb of at least < 10 g/dL.[75]

There is good evidence from one methodologically sound, large multicenter trial that intravenous iron carboxymaltose improves exercise tolerance, quality of life, and exercise duration in patients with chronic, stable systolic heart failure.[33] These results are most applicable to iron deficient patients with NYHA class III heart failure; relatively few patients with milder degrees of heart failure were included. It also may be premature to apply these results to patients with more subtle evidence of relative iron deficiency. Biologic plausibility and test of concept studies suggest iron replacement could play a role in improving symptoms of heart failure even when, theoretically, iron stores are adequate because symptoms may be related to a functional misuse of iron rather than absolute deficiency.[4] Nevertheless, though the criteria used to define iron deficiency were fairly broad, most patients enrolled in the FAIR HF trial had evidence of more advanced iron deficiency and limited iron stores. Finally, though these results are encouraging and have the potential to influence treatment of heart failure, the long-term health and cost implications of this are uncertain, and harms have not been more widely assessed.

Despite a paucity of data to support this contention, for decades, many physicians adhered to the "10/30 rule," transfusing patients with hemoglobin under 10 g/dL and hematocrit under 30 percent for perceived safety reasons.[76] In recent years, the recognition of immunomodulatory effects from leukocyte contamination and changes in RBCs with storage that impair oxygen exchange have led to increased scrutiny of RBC transfusion practice, culminating in the TRICC trial. After its publication, there was widespread adoption of more restrictive transfusion standards. However, because oxygen extraction is already maximized in the coronary circulation, concern has remained that patients with fixed coronary stenoses, who cannot increase blood flow to enhance oxygen delivery, will be more susceptible to ischemia in the setting of anemia and, therefore, should generally be transfused to a higher target than the general population. Often, this continues to be a hemoglobin of 10 g/dL.

In the perioperative literature, accumulating evidence from randomized controlled trials supports use of a conservative hemoglobin trigger no higher than 8 g/dL among heart disease patients in the intra- and postoperative setting. The results of the FOCUS trial, by far the largest study to investigate transfusion use in heart disease with over 2,000 enrolled patients, have thus far been released only in abstract form, but it found no difference in mortality, ability to walk across a room unaided, falls, or readmissions with transfusion at a threshold of 8 versus 10 g/dL.[69] While they have some methodological weaknesses, four randomized controlled trials in cardiac surgery, one additional study in hip fracture, and one trial in vascular surgery all were consistent in finding no difference in mortality or other health outcomes with more restrictive use of transfusion.[63-68] No similar trial has been conducted in the general surgery population.

The data from observational studies in the perioperative setting are congruent with the results from randomized controlled trials. In non-cardiac surgery cohorts, transfusion did not appear to offer any protection.[41, 68, 70] We chose to exclude cardiac surgery observational cohorts from our review; nevertheless, in 13 out of 14 such studies aggregated in two prior reviews, the primary results suggested increased risk of adverse clinical events, and the fourteenth was neutral.[77, 78]

No definitive conclusions about best transfusion practice in heart disease outside of the perioperative setting can be drawn from the evidence from randomized controlled trials. The TRICC subgroup analysis found no significant difference in survival between restrictive and liberal transfusion groups, but mortality was slightly lower in the liberally transfused group, a trend opposite of that noted in the overall population or any other studied subgroup.[39] In any case, it is difficult to extrapolate from this critically ill population, where the mean APACHE II score was 23, most patients were mechanically ventilated, and many had noncardiac primary diagnoses. Meanwhile, the CRIT trial suggests that transfusion leads to heart failure exacerbations in ACS patients but was too small to properly evaluate for any effect on survival or recurrent myocardial ischemia.[40] Results from the in-progress MINT trial may shed some light, but it is also small and designed only as a pilot, with the plan for a large scale follow-up trial.

Despite the limitations inherent to their design, several themes emerged in our review of the observational data that can potentially help to guide practice: 1) the evidence strongly suggests that transfusion has no benefit and may be harmful in patients with heart disease and hemoglobin > 10 g/dL; 2) outcomes do not appear to improve with transfusion in non-ST-elevation ACS patients with hemoglobin levels down to the 8 – 9 g/dL range; 3) transfusion is consistently associated with higher mortality risk in the unselected PCI population, across multiple studies with mean nadir hemoglobins of 8 – 9 g/dL; and 4) the elevated risk in the PCI population is seen in patients with anemia related or unrelated to bleeding but may be higher in the non-bleeding anemic population. There is no evidence to guide decision-making in the stable coronary disease population, and the two studies in decompensated heart failure have conflicting results.

One of the larger questions remains: at what hemoglobin threshold does transfusion become protective in ACS patients (i.e., the risks of anemia exceed the hazards of transfusion)? Wu et al. found that transfused AMI patients had lower adjusted mortality than nontransfused patients at any hemoglobin level under 10-11 g/dL,[59] and Sabatine et al. noted that STEMI patients appeared to have lower cardiovascular mortality if they received PRBCs at a hemoglobin below a threshold of 12 g/dL.[57] In contrast, Sabatine found increased risk of major adverse cardiac events in NSTE-ACS patients who received transfusion at any hemoglobin level; and Rao et al. found no benefit to transfusion in NSTE-ACS down to hemoglobin of ~7 g/dL, and a substantially increased risk of death with transfusion above hemoglobin of 10 g/dL.[52] One other study found a significantly reduced risk of death at six months in AMI patients transfused at hemoglobin < 8 g/dL,[58] and two noted non-significant trends toward improved survival in NSTE-ACS with transfusion at a hemoglobin below 8 – 9 g/dL.[54, 55] All three studies found higher adjusted mortality in patients transfused above the 8 – 9 g/dL hemoglobin threshold.

Why might the identified hemoglobin thresholds differ across studies? In particular, can we explain the outlier findings by Wu and Sabatine that transfusion may be beneficial above a hemoglobin of 10 g/dL? The patients in the Wu study were generally older than in other trials, with potentially greater comorbidities (having not been screened for a clinical trial), and had lower rates of exposure to red blood cells. In contrast to many of the other studies, the Wu study relied on claims data with limited granularity. For example, the study grouped patients according to baseline anemia and did not examine how the development of anemia during hospitalization or the timing of transfusion affected outcomes. Though they excluded patients with major bleeding, it is almost certain that mean hemoglobin fell over the course of hospitalization; thus, their results, stratified by admission hemoglobin, would seem to overestimate any potential nadir hemoglobin threshold below which transfusion may be beneficial. Wu also excluded patients who underwent CABG, and fewer patients in the Wu study had PCI or reperfusion therapy. In theory, revascularized/reperfused patients may be more tolerant of severe anemia than their conservatively managed counterparts, since they can increase myocardial oxygen delivery through augmentation of blood flow without the need for PRBCs.

The Sabatine study results suggest that STEMI patients, who suffer abrupt and complete occlusion of a coronary artery, may have a lower tolerance for anemia than NSTE-ACS patients and thus benefit more from transfusion, even to a hemoglobin of 12 g/dL. However, like Wu et al., they used admission hemoglobin in their study, so their results likely inflate the threshold hemoglobin nadir. Moreover, several other studies that included STEMI patients primarily or exclusively did not find any evidence of benefit from transfusion.[50, 51, 56, 58] PCI rates were generally higher in these studies, however, which again might explain the difference.

As noted, aside from inconsistency of results, the major limitation of this body of observational studies is selection bias, namely, confounding by indication.[79] In other words, because of the observational nature of these studies, the decision to transfuse patients was based on clinical judgment which, in turn, would be naturally influenced by severity of illness, symptoms, and observation of bleeding. Indeed, the studies show that the groups who were transfused more aggressively were more severely ill. Additionally, bleeding rates did vary substantially across studies but were inconsistently reported; one might reasonably expect that the risk-benefit balance of red blood cell transfusion would change in the setting of bleeding compared to stable blood volume. Despite, in some cases, the very careful propensity adjustment, the possibility of residual confounding remains and renders this a fairly tenuous evidence base.

Perhaps in part because of the conflicting results, there is continued widespread variation in RBC transfusion practices, highlighting the need for more definitive guidance from large controlled clinical trials examining the comparative benefits of liberal and conservative transfusion strategies in patients with heart disease. Of note, the CRIT trial could not enroll their goal of 92 patients in over six years of active recruitment; it is not clear why there were difficulties with recruitment, but this raises concerns about the feasibility of a large scale trial. There is increasing evidence as well that freshly collected units may be safer and more effective than PRBCs stored for longer periods;[45, 80] future studies should also look specifically at the comparative benefits/risks of transfusion of fresh RBCs in the heart disease population.

CLINICAL APPLICATIONS

Clinicians encounter anemia in many different types of patients with heart disease, and may need to understand how the overall evidence base for anemia treatment pertains to the patient in front of them. Here we summarize how the data presented previously might apply to different common clinical scenarios:

1. Outpatient with stable NYHA class III congestive heart failure, ferritin of 50 μg/dL and a Hgb of 10g/dL

   Intravenous iron supplementation could be considered to improve symptoms, but there is no consistent good-quality evidence at this time to support the use of ESAs or blood transfusions in this patient. The use of iron could even be considered if this patient had a normal hemoglobin. Of note, the data supporting IV iron comes largely from one trial, albeit a well-conducted one, that reported only short-term quality of life and exercise tolerance outcomes.[33] Furthermore, the use of IV iron would be unsupported if this patient had milder heart failure symptoms or if the ferritin were normal given that there were few such patients included in the trial. Though a number of trials have examined the use of ESAs for patients similar to this, they do not convincingly show a consistent benefit and there may be important harms, especially if this patient had advanced kidney disease. A larger ongoing trial of

ESA use should better clarify their role in this type of patient. There are no trials of blood transfusions applicable to this patient.

2. Outpatient with stable NYHA class III congestive heart failure, end stage renal disease on hemodialysis, and Hgb 9 g/dL

    The decision to use ESAs would be based largely on this patient's comorbid kidney disease rather than the heart disease itself. The once common practice of using ESAs to raise hemoglobin in patients with advanced chronic kidney disease has been undermined by recent large-scale trials, and new FDA recommendations suggest use of ESAs only for patients with Hgb < 10 g/dL, and with as low a dose necessary to obviate blood transfusion. Three of these trials included substantial proportions of heart disease patients and found no benefit and possible serious harms from ESAs titrated to normal or near-normal hemoglobin.[13, 26, 30] The benefit of titrating ESAs to lower hemoglobin targets in patients with heart disease and advanced kidney disease remains unexplored. There are no studies of iron supplementation or blood transfusion that would apply to this patient.

3. Hospitalized patient with decompensated heart failure and Hgb 9 g/dL

    There is no data to guide the use of ESAs or iron in this patient. It is noteworthy that nearly all of the ESA and iron trials reviewed would have excluded patients like this with decompensated disease. Two observational studies of blood transfusions in patients hospitalized with CHF found conflicting results and do not convincingly support routine transfusion of patients like this, though the evidence base is very limited.

4. Patient with acute coronary syndrome and Hgb 9 g/dL

    There is very little good direct evidence to guide whether or not to administer blood transfusions in this patient. One older trial of critically ill patients with cardiovascular disease found that patients transfused more aggressively (Hgb threshold 10 g/dL) did no better than those transfused less aggressively (threshold 7 g/dL). A small recent trial suggested a more aggressive strategy may actually be harmful in patients with acute coronary syndrome. Many observational studies in patients with ACS have found conflicting results, though the majority of them suggest increased harms associated with transfusions certainly above Hgb 10g/dL and in some cases, above Hgb > 8 g/dL, especially in patients who have undergone PCI.

    No trials have evaluated iron in patients with ACS.

5. Outpatient with chronic stable angina and Hgb 8 g/dL

    There is no good evidence that directly applies to this patient. However, a large study of patients with ESRD and heart disease, many of whom had a history of angina, showed ESAs titrated to a normal hemoglobin did not reduce the incidence of angina requiring hospitalization and was associated with increased thrombotic events and higher mortality.[26] Though patients in this study also received IV iron, there are no studies of IV iron alone in patients with chronic stable angina, nor are there studies examining blood transfusions.

6. Patient admitted with a hip fracture awaiting surgery who has known, stable CHD and anemia with a Hgb of 9 g/dL

There is no evidence that transfusing such patients above a hemoglobin of 8 g/dL improves outcomes. Data from one large randomized controlled trial and a smaller pilot study found no benefit of transfusing patients to a target hemoglobin of 10 g/dL compared to 8 g/dL. There is no data which addresses the use of ESAs or iron in such patients.

LIMITATIONS

Because our review was focused on patient-centered health outcomes, we did not include physiologic surrogates of exercise tolerance such as Vo2 max. In excluding such outcomes, we could have missed evidence of benefit on proximal outcomes. The largest ESA trials by far are those of patients with advanced renal disease and comorbid heart disease. We felt it important to include these studies given the large proportion of heart disease patients with comorbid chronic kidney disease and the potential harms these studies underscore. However, we acknowledge the limited applicability of these results to many patients with heart failure. The inclusion of observational studies in our review of the efficacy of blood transfusions may risk overstating the depth of the evidence base when, in fact, there is little trial data to guide practice and the risk of bias in the observational studies is likely too high to make them a reliable source of evidence to guide decision-making. Nevertheless, we felt the inclusion of such studies would allow greater transparency of the types of studies that are, de facto, currently guiding practice.

FUTURE STUDIES

Ongoing studies such as RED-HF should be able to more clearly define whether or not there is a role for ESAs in the treatment of anemic heart failure patients. If the study results are positive, there may be a need for future studies comparing the relative benefits of ESAs and iron in heart failure patients. Given that most ESA studies were conducted in patients with systolic dysfunction but a large proportion of CHF patients have preserved systolic function, future studies should clarify the role of ESAs in patients with preserved systolic function. There should be more studies of anemic patients with ischemic heart disease. Future studies should better clarify the influence of chronic kidney disease on the effectiveness of various anemia treatments. Rather than the very high hemoglobin targets trials to date have examined in patients with advanced kidney disease, future studies may consider the value of more moderate hemoglobin targets given the remaining uncertainty for patients with moderate anemia. There is a pressing need for more trials examining the role of blood transfusions; treatment of patients with stable or decompensated heart failure, as well as patients with stable, asymptomatic or actively symptomatic ischemic heart disease, remains uncertain.

CONCLUSIONS

Anemia is common in patients with heart disease, but the evidence base to date does not convincingly support a role for ESAs for anemia correction. Iron treatment may help ameliorate symptoms over the short-term in patients with symptomatic heart failure. The role of blood transfusions remains understudied and unclear. Table 5 summarizes the evidence on the effectiveness of these therapies according to patient population and outcome.

Table 5. Summary of the Evidence for the Effects of ESAs, Iron and Blood Transfusions for Anemia, by Patient Population and Outcome

Treatment	Outcome	Effect*	GRADE Classification†	Comment
Stable CHF, and no worse than stage 3 CKD				
ESAs	Exercise tolerance and duration	(~)	Moderate	Inconsistent results and methodologic weaknesses in some studies limit the evidence base. Overall, studies with low risk of bias found no significant effect.
	Quality of life	(~)	Low	Infrequent reporting, inconsistent results, the variety of instruments used, and methodologic weaknesses in some studies greatly limit the evidence base.
	Mortality	(~)	Low	Based on mainly small, single center trials with limited power and low event rates.
	Hospitalizations	(~)	Low	Inconsistent results and methodologic weaknesses in some studies limit the evidence base. The two studies with low risk of bias found no significant effect.
	Harms including hypertension, cerebrovascular and thrombotic events	(~)	Low	Based on mainly small, single-center trials with low event rates.
Iron	Exercise tolerance and duration	(+)	Moderate/High	One well-conducted large multicenter trial and two smaller trials found benefit.
	Quality of life	(+)	Moderate/High	One well-conducted large multicenter trial and two smaller trials found benefit.
	Mortality	(~)/(+)	Low	The one large trial showed a trend towards benefit, but was, like the two smaller trials, not powered for this outcome.
	Cardiovascular events	(+)	Moderate	One large multicenter trial found benefit, but follow-up was relatively short.
	Serious harms	(~)	Moderate	Based on one large and two small trials.
Blood transfusions	All outcomes	(0)		No evidence.
Stable CHF, and stage 4 or 5 CKD				
ESAs	Exercise tolerance and duration	(0)		No evidence. Trials including subgroups of CHF patients did not report this outcome separately.
	Quality of life	(~)	Low	One large trial of heart disease patients including large subgroup of CHF patients, but subgroup specific data not available.
	Mortality	(–)	Moderate	Based on two large trials including large numbers with CHF; in one trial the increased risk of mortality was not significant; type and severity of CHF not reported.
	Cardiovascular events	(~)	High	Based on three large trials including large numbers with CHF; type and severity of CHF not reported.
	Venous thrombosis	(–)	Moderate	Based on two large trials including large numbers with CHF; type and severity of CHF not reported; effects of more moderate hemoglobin targets not tested.

Treatment	Outcome	Effect*	GRADE Classification†	Comment
	Hypertension, cerebrovascular events	(−)	Low	Based on one large trial including large numbers with CHF, but CHF subgroup data not separately reported for this outcome.
Iron	All outcomes	(0)		No evidence.
Blood transfusions	All outcomes	(0)		No evidence.
Decompensated CHF				
ESAs	All outcomes	(0)		No evidence.
Iron	All outcomes	(0)		No evidence.
Blood transfusions	Mortality	(−)	Very low	Two observational studies found conflicting results – one showed harm, one a possible benefit.
Stable CHD				
ESAs	Mortality	(−)	Low	One large trial of heart disease patients including large subgroup of CHD patients, but subgroup specific data not available. Patients with ESRD, unclear application to other populations.
	Quality of life	(~)	Low	One large trial of heart disease patients including large subgroup of CHD patients, but subgroup specific data not available. Patients with ESRD, unclear application to other populations.
	Venous thrombosis	(−)	Low	One large trial of heart disease patients including large subgroup of CHD patients, but subgroup specific data not available. Patients with ESRD, unclear application to other populations.
	All other outcomes	(0)		No evidence.
Iron	All outcomes	(0)		No evidence.
Blood transfusions	All outcomes	(0)		No evidence.
Acute coronary syndrome				
ESAs	All outcomes	(0)		No evidence.
Iron	All outcomes	(0)		No evidence.
Blood transfusions	Mortality	(~)	Moderate	Two RCTs, one with limited applicability to non ICU population, showed no benefit from transfusing above Hgb > 10 g/dL. Observational studies in PCI patients consistently showed no benefit and possible harm.
	Cardiovascular events	(~)	Low	Two RCTs found conflicting results: one found harm, a larger trial found no effect. Observational studies did not commonly report this as a separate outcome.
Non-cardiac surgery				
ESAs	All outcomes	(0)		No evidence.
Iron	All outcomes	(0)		No evidence.

Treatment	Outcome	Effect*	GRADE Classification†	Comment
Blood transfusions	Mortality	(~)	Low	One large RCT, but reported only in abstract form and only applicable to hip fracture patients.
Cardiac surgery				
ESAs	All outcomes	(0)		No evidence.
Iron	All outcomes	(0)		No evidence.
Blood transfusions	Mortality	(~)	Moderate	Two large and two small RCTs with some methodologic weaknesses.

GRADE = Grades of Recommendation, Assessment, Development, and Evaluation; ICU = intensive care unit; RCT = randomized controlled trial.

*Effect: (+) benefit; (−) harm; (~) mixed findings/no effect; (0) no evidence.

† GRADE classification: high = further research is very unlikely to change our confidence on the estimate of effect; moderate = further research is likely to have an important impact on our confidence in the estimate of effect and may change the estimate; low = further research is very likely to have an important impact on our confidence in the estimate of effect and is likely to change the estimate; very low = any estimate of effect is very uncertain.

REFERENCES

1. Boyd CM, Leff B, Wolff JL, et al. Informing clinical practice guideline development and implementation: prevalence of coexisting conditions among adults with coronary heart disease. *Journal of the American Geriatrics Society.* May 2011;59(5):797-805.

2. Felker GM, Adams KF, Jr., Gattis WA, O'Connor CM. Anemia as a risk factor and therapeutic target in heart failure. *Journal of the American College of Cardiology.* Sep 1 2004;44(5):959-966.

3. Malyszko J, Bachorzewska-Gajewska H, Levin-Iaina N, et al. Prevalence of chronic kidney disease and anemia in patients with coronary artery disease with normal serum creatinine undergoing percutaneous coronary interventions: relation to New York Heart Association class. *Israel Medical Association Journal: Imaj.* Aug 2010;12(8):489-493.

4. Gonzalez-Costello J, Comin-Colet J. Iron deficiency and anaemia in heart failure: understanding the FAIR-HF trial. *European Journal of Heart Failure.* Nov 2010;12(11):1159-1162.

5. Komajda M, Anker SD, Charlesworth A, et al. The impact of new onset anaemia on morbidity and mortality in chronic heart failure: results from COMET. *European Heart Journal.* Jun 2006;27(12):1440-1446.

6. Kosiborod M, Smith GL, Radford MJ, Foody JM, Krumholz HM. The prognostic importance of anemia in patients with heart failure. *American Journal of Medicine.* Feb 1 2003;114(2):112-119.

7. Silverberg DS, Wexler D, Blum M, et al. The use of subcutaneous erythropoietin and intravenous iron for the treatment of the anemia of severe, resistant congestive heart failure improves cardiac and renal function and functional cardiac class, and markedly reduces hospitalizations. *Journal of the American College of Cardiology.* Jun 2000;35(7):1737-1744.

8. Higgins JPT, Altman DG, editors. Chapter 8: Assessing risk of bias in included studies. In: Higgins JPT, Green S (editors). *Cochrane Handbook for Systematic Reviews of Interventions.* 2008;Version 5.0.1. The Cochrane Collaboration, 2008. Availablefrom www.cochrane-handbook.org.

9. Atkins D, Best D, Briss PA, et al. Grading quality of evidence and strength of recommendations. *BMJ.* Jun 19 2004;328(7454):1490.

10. DerSimonian R, Laird N. Meta-analysis in clinical trials. *Control Clin Trials.* Sep 1986;7(3):177-188.

11. Egger M, Davey Smith G, Schneider M, Minder C. Bias in meta-analysis detected by a simple, graphical test. *BMJ.* Sep 13 1997;315(7109):629-634.

12.   Comin-Colet J, Ruiz S, Cladellas M, Rizzo M, Torres A, Bruguera J. A pilot evaluation of the long-term effect of combined therapy with intravenous iron sucrose and erythropoietin in elderly patients with advanced chronic heart failure and cardio-renal anemia syndrome: influence on neurohormonal activation and clinical outcomes. *Journal of Cardiac Failure.* Nov 2009;15(9):727-735.

13.   Szczech LA, Barnhart HX, Sapp S, et al. A secondary analysis of the CHOIR trial shows that comorbid conditions differentially affect outcomes during anemia treatment. *Kidney International.* Feb 2010;77(3):239-246.

14.   Pfeffer MA, Burdmann EA, Chen C-Y, et al. Baseline characteristics in the Trial to Reduce Cardiovascular Events With Aranesp Therapy (TREAT). *American Journal of Kidney Diseases.* Jul 2009;54(1):59-69.

15.   Palazzuoli A, Silverberg DS, Calabr, et al. Beta-erythropoietin effects on ventricular remodeling, left and right systolic function, pulmonary pressure, and hospitalizations in patients affected with heart failure and anemia. *Journal of Cardiovascular Pharmacology.* Jun 2009;53(6):462-467.

16.   Parissis JT, Kourea K, Andreadou I, et al. Effects of Darbepoetin Alfa on plasma mediators of oxidative and nitrosative stress in anemic patients with chronic heart failure secondary to ischemic or idiopathic dilated cardiomyopathy. *American Journal of Cardiology.* Apr 15 2009;103(8):1134-1138.

17.   Kourea K, Parissis JT, Farmakis D, et al. Effects of darbepoetin-alpha on quality of life and emotional stress in anemic patients with chronic heart failure. *European Journal of Cardiovascular Prevention & Rehabilitation.* Jun 2008;15(3):365-369.

18.   Parissis JT, Kourea K, Panou F, et al. Effects of darbepoetin alpha on right and left ventricular systolic and diastolic function in anemic patients with chronic heart failure secondary to ischemic or idiopathic dilated cardiomyopathy. *American Heart Journal.* Apr 2008;155(4):751.e751-757.

19.   Ghali JK, Anand IS, Abraham WT, et al. Randomized double-blind trial of darbepoetin alfa in patients with symptomatic heart failure and anemia. *Circulation.* Jan 29 2008;117(4):526-535.

20.   Besarab A, Goodkin DA, Nissenson AR, Normal Hematocrit Cardiac Trial A. The normal hematocrit study--follow-up. *New England Journal of Medicine.* Jan 24 2008;358(4):433-434.

21.   Palazzuoli A, Silverberg DS, Iovine F, et al. Effects of beta-erythropoietin treatment on left ventricular remodeling, systolic function, and B-type natriuretic peptide levels in patients with the cardiorenal anemia syndrome. *American Heart Journal.* Oct 2007;154(4):645.e649-615.

22.   van Veldhuisen DJ, Dickstein K, Cohen-Solal A, et al. Randomized, double-blind, placebo-controlled study to evaluate the effect of two dosing regimens of darbepoetin alfa in patients with heart failure and anaemia. *European Heart Journal.* Sep 2007;28(18):2208-2216.

23.   Ponikowski P, Anker SD, Szachniewicz J, et al. Effect of darbepoetin alfa on exercise tolerance in anemic patients with symptomatic chronic heart failure: a randomized, double-blind, placebo-controlled trial. *Journal of the American College of Cardiology.* Feb 20 2007;49(7):753-762.

24.   Mancini DM, Kunavarapu C. Effect of erythropoietin on exercise capacity in anemic patients with advanced heart failure. *Kidney International - Supplement.* Nov 2003(87):S48-52.

25.   Silverberg DS, Wexler D, Sheps D, et al. The effect of correction of mild anemia in severe, resistant congestive heart failure using subcutaneous erythropoietin and intravenous iron: a randomized controlled study. *Journal of the American College of Cardiology.* Jun 1 2001;37(7):1775-1780.

26.   Besarab A, Bolton WK, Browne JK, et al. The effects of normal as compared with low hematocrit values in patients with cardiac disease who are receiving hemodialysis and epoetin. *New England Journal of Medicine.* Aug 27 1998;339(9):584-590.

27.   Bellinghieri G, Savica V, De Gregorio C, De Gregorio G. Use of erythropoietin in ischemic and arrhythmic cardiopathy of hemodialyzed patients. *Contributions to Nephrology.* 1994;106:135-137.

28.   Palazzuoli A, Silverberg D, Iovine F, et al. Erythropoietin improves anemia exercise tolerance and renal function and reduces B-type natriuretic peptide and hospitalization in patients with heart failure and anemia. *American Heart Journal.* Dec 2006;152(6):1096. e1099-1015.

29.   Desai A, Lewis E, Solomon S, McMurray JJV, Pfeffer M. Impact of erythropoiesis-stimulating agents on morbidity and mortality in patients with heart failure: An updated, post-TREAT meta-analysis. *European Journal of Heart Failure.* 2010;12(9):936-942.

30.   Pfeffer MA, Burdmann EA, Chen C-Y, et al. A trial of darbepoetin alfa in type 2 diabetes and chronic kidney disease. *New England Journal of Medicine.* Nov 19 2009;361(21):2019-2032.

31.   Amgen. RED-HF™ Trial - Reduction of Events With Darbepoetin Alfa in Heart Failure Trial. ClinicalTrials.gov identifier: NCT00358215. Ongoing study.

32.   Maurer MS. Anemia in Heart Failure With a Preserved Ejection Fraction (HFPEF). ClinicalTrials.gov Identifier: NCT00286182. Ongoing study.

33.   Anker SD, Comin Colet J, Filippatos G, et al. Ferric carboxymaltose in patients with heart failure and iron deficiency. *New England Journal of Medicine.* Dec 17 2009;361(25):2436-2448.

34.   Toblli JE, Lombra, x00F, a A, Duarte P, Di Gennaro F. Intravenous iron reduces NT-pro-brain natriuretic peptide in anemic patients with chronic heart failure and renal insufficiency. *Journal of the American College of Cardiology.* Oct 23 2007;50(17):1657-1665.

35.   Okonko DO, Grzeslo A, Witkowski T, et al. Effect of intravenous iron sucrose on exercise tolerance in anemic and nonanemic patients with symptomatic chronic heart failure and iron deficiency FERRIC-HF: a randomized, controlled, observer-blinded trial. *Journal of the American College of Cardiology.* Jan 15 2008;51(2):103-112.

36.   Maluenda G, Lemesle G, Ben-Dor I, et al. Value of blood transfusion in patients with a blood hematocrit of 24% to 30% after percutaneous coronary intervention. *American Journal of Cardiology.* Oct 15 2009;104(8):1069-1073.

37.   Maluenda G, Lemesle G, Syed A, et al. Does transfusion for major bleeding after percutaneous coronary intervention impact clinical outcome in patients admitted with normal Hematocrit? *Journal of the American College of Cardiology.* 2009;53(10):A72.

38.   Maluenda G, Lemesle G, Syed A, et al. Should patients who develop anemia (hematocrit (less-than or equal to) 27%) after percutaneous coronary intervention be transfused? *Journal of the American College of Cardiology.* 2009;53(10):A84.

39.   Hebert PC, Yetisir E, Martin C, et al. Is a low transfusion threshold safe in critically ill patients with cardiovascular diseases? *Critical Care Medicine.* Feb 2001;29(2):227-234.

40.   Cooper HA, Rao SV, Greenberg MD, et al. Conservative Versus Liberal Red Cell Transfusion in Acute Myocardial Infarction (the CRIT Randomized Pilot Study). *The American journal of cardiology.* 2011.

41.   Bursi F, Barbieri A, Politi L, et al. Perioperative red blood cell transfusion and outcome in stable patients after elective major vascular surgery. *European Journal of Vascular & Endovascular Surgery.* Mar 2009;37(3):311-318.

42.   Hebert PC, Wells G, Blajchman MA, et al. A multicenter, randomized, controlled clinical trial of transfusion requirements in critical care. Transfusion Requirements in Critical Care Investigators, Canadian Critical Care Trials Group. *New England Journal of Medicine.* Feb 11 1999;340(6):409-417.

43.   Carson JL. Myocardial Ischemia and Transfusion (MINT). ClinicalTrials.gov identifier: NCT01167582. Ongoing study.

44.   Kinnaird TD, Stabile E, Mintz GS, et al. Incidence, predictors, and prognostic implications of bleeding and blood transfusion following percutaneous coronary interventions. *American Journal of Cardiology.* Oct 15 2003;92(8):930-935.

45.   Kim P, Dixon S, Eisenbrey AB, O'Malley B, Boura J, O'Neill W. Impact of acute blood loss anemia and red blood cell transfusion on mortality after percutaneous coronary intervention. *Clinical Cardiology.* Oct 2007;30(10 Suppl 2):II35-43.

46.   Yatskar L, Selzer F, Feit F, et al. Access site hematoma requiring blood transfusion predicts mortality in patients undergoing percutaneous coronary intervention: data from the National Heart, Lung, and Blood Institute Dynamic Registry. *Catheter Cardiovasc Interv.* Jun 1 2007;69(7):961-966.

47.   Doyle BJ, Ting HH, Bell MR, et al. Major femoral bleeding complications after percutaneous coronary intervention: incidence, predictors, and impact on long-term survival among 17,901 patients treated at the Mayo Clinic from 1994 to 2005. *Jacc: Cardiovascular Interventions.* Apr 2008;1(2):202-209.

48.   Chase AJ, Fretz EB, Warburton WP, et al. Association of the arterial access site at angioplasty with transfusion and mortality: the M.O.R.T.A.L study (Mortality benefit Of Reduced Transfusion after percutaneous coronary intervention via the Arm or Leg). *Heart.* Aug 2008;94(8):1019-1025.

49.   Jani SM, Smith DE, Share D, et al. Blood transfusion and in-hospital outcomes in anemic patients with myocardial infarction undergoing percutaneous coronary intervention. *Clinical Cardiology.* Oct 2007;30(10 Suppl 2):II49-56.

50.   Jolicoeur EM, O'Neill WW, Hellkamp A, et al. Transfusion and mortality in patients with ST-segment elevation myocardial infarction treated with primary percutaneous coronary intervention. *European Heart Journal.* Nov 2009;30(21):2575-2583.

51.   Nikolsky E, Mehran R, Sadeghi HM, et al. Prognostic impact of blood transfusion after primary angioplasty for acute myocardial infarction: analysis from the CADILLAC (Controlled Abciximab and Device Investigation to Lower Late Angioplasty Complications) Trial. *Jacc: Cardiovascular Interventions.* Jul 2009;2(7):624-632.

52.   Rao SV, Jollis JG, Harrington RA, et al. Relationship of blood transfusion and clinical outcomes in patients with acute coronary syndromes. *Journal of the American Medical Association.* 2004;292(13):1555-1562.

53.   Yang X, Alexander KP, Chen AY, et al. The implications of blood transfusions for patients with non-ST-segment elevation acute coronary syndromes: results from the CRUSADE National Quality Improvement Initiative. *Journal of the American College of Cardiology.* Oct 18 2005;46(8):1490-1495.

54.   Singla I, Zahid M, Good CB, Macioce A, Sonel AF. Impact of blood transfusions in patients presenting with anemia and suspected acute coronary syndrome. *American Journal of Cardiology.* Apr 15 2007;99(8):1119-1121.

55.   Alexander KP, Chen AY, Wang TY, et al. Transfusion practice and outcomes in non-ST-segment elevation acute coronary syndromes. *American Heart Journal.* Jun 2008;155(6):1047-1053.

56.   Shishehbor MH, Madhwal S, Rajagopal V, et al. Impact of blood transfusion on short- and long-term mortality in patients with ST-segment elevation myocardial infarction. *Jacc: Cardiovascular Interventions.* Jan 2009;2(1):46-53.

57.   Sabatine MS, Morrow DA, Giugliano RP, et al. Association of hemoglobin levels with clinical outcomes in acute coronary syndromes. *Circulation.* Apr 26 2005;111(16):2042-2049.

58.   Aronson D, Dann EJ, Bonstein L, et al. Impact of red blood cell transfusion on clinical outcomes in patients with acute myocardial infarction. *American Journal of Cardiology.* Jul 15 2008;102(2):115-119.

59.   Wu WC, Rathore SS, Wang Y, Radford MJ, Krumholz HM. Blood transfusion in elderly patients with acute myocardial infarction. *New England Journal of Medicine.* 2001;345(17):1230-1236.

60.   Aggarwal C, Panza JA, Cooper HA, Aggarwal C, Panza JA, Cooper HA. Does the relation between red blood cell transfusion and mortality vary according to transfusion indication? A case-control study among patients with acute coronary syndromes. *Coron Artery Dis.* May 2011;22(3):194-198.

61.   Garty M, Cohen E, Zuchenko A, et al. Blood transfusion for acute decompensated heart failure--friend or foe? *American Heart Journal.* Oct 2009;158(4):653-658.

62.   Kao DP, Kreso E, Fonarow GC, et al. Characteristics and outcomes among heart failure patients with anemia and renal insufficiency with and without blood transfusions (public discharge data from California 2000-2006). *American Journal of Cardiology.* Jan 2011;107(1):69-73.

63.   Weisel RD, Charlesworth DC, Mickleborough LL, et al. Limitations of blood conservation. *Journal of Thoracic & Cardiovascular Surgery.* Jul 1984;88(1):26-38.

64.   Johnson RG, Thurer RL, Kruskall MS, et al. Comparison of two transfusion strategies after elective operations for myocardial revascularization. *Journal of Thoracic & Cardiovascular Surgery.* Aug 1992;104(2):307-314.

65.   Bracey AW, Radovancevic R, Riggs SA, et al. Lowering the hemoglobin threshold for transfusion in coronary artery bypass procedures: effect on patient outcome. *Transfusion.* Oct 1999;39(10):1070-1077.

66.   Hajjar LA, Vincent JL, Galas FR, et al. Transfusion requirements after cardiac surgery: the TRACS randomized controlled trial. *JAMA.* Oct 13 2010;304(14):1559-1567.

67.   Bush RL, Pevec WC, Holcroft JW. A prospective, randomized trial limiting perioperative red blood cell transfusions in vascular patients. *American Journal of Surgery.* Aug 1997;174(2):143-148.

68.   Carson JL, Terrin ML, Barton FB, et al. A pilot randomized trial comparing symptomatic vs. hemoglobin-level-driven red blood cell transfusions following hip fracture. *Transfusion.* Jun 1998;38(6):522-529.

69.   Carson JL, Terrin ML, Magaziner J, Sanders D, Cook DR, Hildebrand K. Transfusion trigger trial for functional outcomes in cardiovascular patients undergoing surgical hip fracture repair (FOCUS): The principal results. *Blood.* 2009;114(22).

70. Glance LG, Dick AW, Mukamel DB, et al. Association between intraoperative blood transfusion and mortality and morbidity in patients undergoing noncardiac surgery. *Anesthesiology.* Feb 2011;114(2):283-292.

71. Hebert PC, Wells G, Tweeddale M, et al. Does transfusion practice affect mortality in critically ill patients? Transfusion Requirements in Critical Care (TRICC) Investigators and the Canadian Critical Care Trials Group. *Am J Respir Crit Care Med.* May 1997;155(5):1618-1623.

72. Ngo K, Kotecha D, Walters JA, et al. Erythropoiesis-stimulating agents for anaemia in chronic heart failure patients. *Cochrane Database of Systematic Reviews.* 2010(1):CD007613.

73. Palmer SC, Navaneethan SD, Craig JC, et al. Meta-analysis: erythropoiesis-stimulating agents in patients with chronic kidney disease. *Annals of Internal Medicine.* Jul 6 2010;153(1):23-33.

74. Agency for Healthcare Research and Quality. Comparative Effectiveness of Epoetin and Darbepoetin for Managing Anemia in Patients Undergoing Cancer Treatment - Update DRAFT. *AHRQ Comparative Effectiveness Review.* In progress.

75. U.S. Food and Drug Administration. FDA Drug Safety Communication: Modified dosing recommendations to improve the safe use of Erythropoiesis-Stimulating Agents (ESAs) in chronic kidney disease Accessed 7/29/2011 at http://www.fda.gov/Drugs/DrugSafety/ucm259639.htm#.TjNK6A-AqfM.email.

76. Wang JK, Klein HG. Red blood cell transfusion in the treatment and management of anaemia: the search for the elusive transfusion trigger. *Vox Sanguinis.* Jan 2010;98(1):2-11.

77. Gerber DR. Transfusion of packed red blood cells in patients with ischemic heart disease. *Critical Care Medicine.* Apr 2008;36(4):1068-1074.

78. Marik PE, Corwin HL. Efficacy of red blood cell transfusion in the critically ill: a systematic review of the literature. *Critical Care Medicine.* Sep 2008;36(9):2667-2674.

79. Norris S, Atkins D, Bruening W, et al. Selecting observational studies for comparing medical interventions. In: Agency for Healthcare Research and Quality. Methods Guide for Comparative Effectiveness Reviews. Rockville, MD. Available at: http://www.effectivehealthcare.ahrq.gov/ehc/products/196/454/MethodsGuideNorris_06042010.pdf 2010.

80. Robinson SD, Janssen C, Fretz EB, et al. Red blood cell storage duration and mortality in patients undergoing percutaneous coronary intervention. *American Heart Journal.* May 2010;159(5):876-881.

81. Carson JL, Duff A, Berlin JA, et al. Perioperative blood transfusion and postoperative mortality. *JAMA.* Jan 21 1998;279(3):199-205.

APPENDIX A. SEARCH STRATEGY

anemia	anemia
	anaemia
	anemia/
congestive heart failure/ coronary heart disease/ ischemic heart disease	cardiac failure
	chf
	congestive heart failure
	coronary heart disease
	ischemic heart disease
	heart failure/
	coronary disease/
	myocardial ischemia/
Erythropoiesis-stimulating agents	anti-anaemi*
	antianaemi*
	antianemi*
	anti-anemi*
	aranesp
	darbepoetin
	darbepoietin
	darbopoetin
	epo
	epoetin
	epogen
	epoietin
	eprex
	Erythopoiesis-stimulating agents
	erythropoesis
	erythropoetin
	erythropoiesis
	erythropoietin
	ESA
	ESAs
	hematinics
	neorecormon
	nesp
	procrit
	recormon
	rheupo
	erythropoetin/
Iron - IV or PO	ferric
	ferrous
	iron
	iron/
red blood cell transfusion	red blood cell transfusion
	Erythrocyte Transfusion/
benefits	

harms	safe
	safety
	side-effect*
	undesirable effect*
	treatment emergent
	tolerability
	toxicity
	adverse adj2 (effect or effects or reaction or reactions or event or events or outcome or outcomes)
	/adverse effects
	/poisoning
	/toxicity
	/chemically induced
	/contraindications
	/complications
	thromboembolism
	thromboembolism/
threshold hemoglobin value	threshold hemoglobin value
RCT	1 randomized controlled trial.pt. 2 controlled clinical trial.pt. 3 randomized.ab. 4 placebo.ab. 5 drug therapy.fs. 6 randomly.ab. 7 trial.ab. 8 groups.ab 9 1 or 2 or 3 or 4 or 5 or 6 or 7 or 8 10 exp animals/ not humans.sh. 11 9 not 10 [Cochrane's Highly Sensitive Search Strategy for identifying randomized trials in MEDLINE: sensitivity-maximizing version (2008 revision); Ovid format]
human	not (not human)

Databases: MEDLINE, Cochrane, EMBASE

ESA Benefits – search strategy

Database(s):**Ovid MEDLINE® and Ovid OLDMEDLINE®** 1947 to November Week 1 2010, **Ovid MEDLINE® In-Process & Other Non-Indexed Citations** November 11, 2010

#	Searches	Results
1	anemia.mp. or exp Anemia/	149879
2	anaemia.mp.	22339
3	1 or 2	157901
4	cardiac failure.mp. or exp Heart Failure/	77416
5	chf.mp.	8843
6	congestive heart failure.mp.	28353
7	coronary heart disease.mp. or exp Coronary Disease/	177123
8	ischemic heart disease.mp. or exp Myocardial Ischemia/	321932
9	4 or 5 or 6 or 7 or 8	407842

10	3 and 9	2677
11	anti-anaemi*.mp. [mp=title, original title, abstract, name of substance word, subject heading word, unique identifier]	33
12	antianaemi*.mp. [mp=title, original title, abstract, name of substance word, subject heading word, unique identifier]	30
13	antianemi*.mp. [mp=title, original title, abstract, name of substance word, subject heading word, unique identifier]	174
14	anti-anemi*.mp. [mp=title, original title, abstract, name of substance word, subject heading word, unique identifier]	94
15	aranesp.mp. [mp=title, original title, abstract, name of substance word, subject heading word, unique identifier]	83
16	exp Erythropoietin/ or darbepoetin.mp.	18912
17	darbepoietin.mp.	43
18	darbopoetin.mp. [mp=title, original title, abstract, name of substance word, subject heading word, unique identifier]	3
19	epo.mp. [mp=title, original title, abstract, name of substance word, subject heading word, unique identifier]	7585
20	epoetin.mp. [mp=title, original title, abstract, name of substance word, subject heading word, unique identifier]	2037
21	epogen.mp. [mp=title, original title, abstract, name of substance word, subject heading word, unique identifier]	61
22	epoietin.mp. [mp=title, original title, abstract, name of substance word, subject heading word, unique identifier]	51
23	eprex.mp. [mp=title, original title, abstract, name of substance word, subject heading word, unique identifier]	126
24	erythropoesis.mp. [mp=title, original title, abstract, name of substance word, subject heading word, unique identifier]	81
25	erythropoetin.mp. [mp=title, original title, abstract, name of substance word, subject heading word, unique identifier]	164
26	erythropoiesis.mp. [mp=title, original title, abstract, name of substance word, subject heading word, unique identifier]	15771
27	erythropoietin.mp. [mp=title, original title, abstract, name of substance word, subject heading word, unique identifier]	23192
28	ESA.mp. [mp=title, original title, abstract, name of substance word, subject heading word, unique identifier]	1138
29	ESAs.mp. [mp=title, original title, abstract, name of substance word, subject heading word, unique identifier]	475
30	hematinics.mp. [mp=title, original title, abstract, name of substance word, subject heading word, unique identifier]	2350
31	neorecormon.mp. [mp=title, original title, abstract, name of substance word, subject heading word, unique identifier]	31
32	nesp.mp. [mp=title, original title, abstract, name of substance word, subject heading word, unique identifier]	73
33	procrit.mp. [mp=title, original title, abstract, name of substance word, subject heading word, unique identifier]	33
34	recormon.mp. [mp=title, original title, abstract, name of substance word, subject heading word, unique identifier]	30
35	Erythropoiesis-stimulating agent.mp. [mp=title, original title, abstract, name of substance word, subject heading word, unique identifier]	152
36	11 or 12 or 13 or 14 or 15 or 16 or 17 or 18 or 19 or 20 or 21 or 22 or 23 24 or 25 or 26 or 27 or 28 or 29 or 30 or 31 or 32 or 33 or 34 or 35	37740

37	randomized controlled trial.pt.	305853
38	controlled clinical trial.pt.	83372
39	randomized.ab.	218942
40	placebo.ab.	127996
41	drug therapy.fs.	1433066
42	randomly.ab.	161893
43	trial.ab.	227198
44	groups.ab.	1067718
45	37 or 38 or 39 or 40 or 41 or 42 or 43 or 44	2717428
46	exp animals/ not humans.sh.	3609973
47	45 not 46	2313774
48	10 and 36 and 47	225

ESA Benefits – search strategy, continued

Database(s):EBM Reviews - Cochrane Central Register of Controlled Trials 4th Quarter 2010
Date searched 11/15/10

#	Searches	Results
1	anemia.mp. or exp Anemia/	4561
2	anaemia.mp.	985
3	1 or 2	5004
4	cardiac failure.mp. or exp Heart Failure/	4150
5	chf.mp.	1152
6	congestive heart failure.mp.	2523
7	coronary heart disease.mp. or exp Coronary Disease/	9300
8	ischemic heart disease.mp. or exp Myocardial Ischemia/	17485
9	4 or 5 or 6 or 7 or 8	23230
10	3 and 9	96
11	anti-anaemi*.mp. [mp=title, original title, abstract, mesh headings, heading words, keyword]	0
12	antianaemi*.mp. [mp=title, original title, abstract, mesh headings, heading words, keyword]	1
13	antianemi*.mp. [mp=title, original title, abstract, mesh headings, heading words, keyword]	16
14	anti-anemi*.mp. [mp=title, original title, abstract, mesh headings, heading words, keyword]	5
15	aranesp.mp. [mp=title, original title, abstract, mesh headings, heading words, keyword]	25
16	exp Erythropoietin/ or darbepoetin.mp.	1291
17	darbepoietin.mp.	9
18	darbopoetin.mp. [mp=title, original title, abstract, mesh headings, heading words, keyword]	9
19	epo.mp. [mp=title, original title, abstract, mesh headings, heading words, keyword]	602
20	epoetin.mp. [mp=title, original title, abstract, mesh headings, heading words, keyword]	603
21	epogen.mp. [mp=title, original title, abstract, mesh headings, heading words, keyword]	2
22	epoietin.mp. [mp=title, original title, abstract, mesh headings, heading words, keyword]	18
23	eprex.mp. [mp=title, original title, abstract, mesh headings, heading words, keyword]	22
24	erythropoesis.mp. [mp=title, original title, abstract, mesh headings, heading words, keyword]	5
25	erythropoetin.mp. [mp=title, original title, abstract, mesh headings, heading words, keyword]	32
26	erythropoiesis.mp. [mp=title, original title, abstract, mesh headings, heading words, keyword]	449
27	erythropoietin.mp. [mp=title, original title, abstract, mesh headings, heading words, keyword]	1903
28	ESA.mp. [mp=title, original title, abstract, mesh headings, heading words, keyword]	51
29	ESAs.mp. [mp=title, original title, abstract, mesh headings, heading words, keyword]	18
30	hematinics.mp. [mp=title, original title, abstract, mesh headings, heading words, keyword]	398
31	neorecormon.mp. [mp=title, original title, abstract, mesh headings, heading words, keyword]	19
32	nesp.mp. [mp=title, original title, abstract, mesh headings, heading words, keyword]	23

33	procrit.mp. [mp=title, original title, abstract, mesh headings, heading words, keyword]	13
34	recormon.mp. [mp=title, original title, abstract, mesh headings, heading words, keyword]	7
35	Erythropoiesis-stimulating agent.mp. [mp=title, original title, abstract, mesh headings, heading words, keyword]	28
36	11 or 12 or 13 or 14 or 15 or 16 or 17 or 18 or 19 or 20 or 21 or 22 or 23 or 24 or 25 or 26 or 27 or 28 or 29 or 30 or 31 or 32 or 33 or 34 or 35	2764
37	randomized controlled trial.pt.	284694
38	controlled clinical trial.pt.	79466
39	randomized.ab.	147977
40	placebo.ab.	100112
41	randomly.ab.	76867
42	trial.ab.	102732
43	groups.ab.	156434
44	37 or 38 or 39 or 40 or 41 or 42 or 43	419005
45	10 and 36 and 44	33

ESA Benefits – search strategy, continued
Database: **EMBASE**
Date searched 11/15/10

#	Query	Results
11	#7 AND #10	105
10	#8 OR #9	346115
9	random$ OR factorial$ OR crossover$ OR cross AND over$ OR 'cross over$' OR placebo$ OR doubl$ AND adj AND blind$ OR single$ AND adj AND blind$ OR assign$ OR allocat$ OR volunteer$ AND [embase]/lim	40406
8	'crossover procedure'/exp OR 'double blind procedure'/exp OR 'randomized controlled trial'/exp OR 'single blind procedure'/exp	310032
7	#5 AND #6	1015
6	'anti anami$' OR antianaemi$ OR antianemi$ AND o$r AND 'anti anemi$' OR 'aranesp'/exp OR 'darbepoetin'/exp OR 'darbepoietin'/exp OR 'darbopoetin'/exp OR epo OR 'epoetin'/exp OR 'epogen'/exp OR 'epoietin'/exp OR 'eprex'/exp OR 'erythopoiesis stimulating' AND agents OR erythropoesis OR erythropoetin OR 'erythropoiesis'/exp OR 'erythropoietin'/exp OR esa OR esas OR 'hematinics'/exp OR 'neorecormon'/exp OR 'nesp'/exp OR 'procrit'/exp OR 'recormon'/exp OR rheupo AND [embase]/lim	70423
5	#1 AND #4	5587
4	#2 OR #3	376323
3	'heart failure'/exp OR 'coronary artery disease'/exp	352502
2	cardiac AND failure OR chf OR congestive AND 'heart'/exp AND failure OR coronary AND 'heart'/exp AND 'disease'/exp OR ischemic AND 'heart'/exp AND 'disease'/exp AND [embase]/lim	43081
1	'anemia'/exp AND [embase]/lim	141383

ESA harms – search strategy
Database(s):**Ovid MEDLINE® and Ovid OLDMEDLINE®** 1947 to November Week 1 2010, **Ovid MEDLINE® In-Process & Other Non-Indexed Citations** November 11, 2010

#	Searches	Results
1	anemia.mp. or exp Anemia/	149879
2	anaemia.mp.	22339
3	1 or 2	157901

4	cardiac failure.mp. or exp Heart Failure/	77416
5	chf.mp.	8843
6	congestive heart failure.mp.	28353
7	coronary heart disease.mp. or exp Coronary Disease/	177123
8	ischemic heart disease.mp. or exp Myocardial Ischemia/	321932
9	4 or 5 or 6 or 7 or 8	407842
10	3 and 9	2677
11	anti-anaemi*.mp. [mp=title, original title, abstract, name of substance word, subject heading word, unique identifier]	33
12	antianaemi*.mp. [mp=title, original title, abstract, name of substance word, subject heading word, unique identifier]	30
13	antianemi*.mp. [mp=title, original title, abstract, name of substance word, subject heading word, unique identifier]	174
14	anti-anemi*.mp. [mp=title, original title, abstract, name of substance word, subject heading word, unique identifier]	94
15	aranesp.mp. [mp=title, original title, abstract, name of substance word, subject heading word, unique identifier]	83
16	exp Erythropoietin/ or darbepoetin.mp.	18912
17	darbepoietin.mp.	43
18	darbopoetin.mp. [mp=title, original title, abstract, name of substance word, subject heading word, unique identifier]	3
19	epo.mp. [mp=title, original title, abstract, name of substance word, subject heading word, unique identifier]	7585
20	epoetin.mp. [mp=title, original title, abstract, name of substance word, subject heading word, unique identifier]	2037
21	epogen.mp. [mp=title, original title, abstract, name of substance word, subject heading word, unique identifier]	61
22	epoietin.mp. [mp=title, original title, abstract, name of substance word, subject heading word, unique identifier]	51
23	eprex.mp. [mp=title, original title, abstract, name of substance word, subject heading word, unique identifier]	126
24	erythropoesis.mp. [mp=title, original title, abstract, name of substance word, subject heading word, unique identifier]	81
25	erythropoetin.mp. [mp=title, original title, abstract, name of substance word, subject heading word, unique identifier]	164
26	erythropoiesis.mp. [mp=title, original title, abstract, name of substance word, subject heading word, unique identifier]	15771
27	erythropoietin.mp. [mp=title, original title, abstract, name of substance word, subject heading word, unique identifier]	23192
28	ESA.mp. [mp=title, original title, abstract, name of substance word, subject heading word, unique identifier]	1138
29	ESAs.mp. [mp=title, original title, abstract, name of substance word, subject heading word, unique identifier]	475
30	hematinics.mp. [mp=title, original title, abstract, name of substance word, subject heading word, unique identifier]	2350
31	neorecormon.mp. [mp=title, original title, abstract, name of substance word, subject heading word, unique identifier]	31
32	nesp.mp. [mp=title, original title, abstract, name of substance word, subject heading word, unique identifier]	73
33	procrit.mp. [mp=title, original title, abstract, name of substance word, subject heading word, unique identifier]	33

34	recormon.mp. [mp=title, original title, abstract, name of substance word, subject heading word, unique identifier]	30
35	Erythropoiesis-stimulating agent.mp. [mp=title, original title, abstract, name of substance word, subject heading word, unique identifier]	152
36	11 or 12 or 13 or 14 or 15 or 16 or 17 or 18 or 19 or 20 or 21 or 22 or 23 or 24 or 25 or 26 or 27 or 28 or 29 or 30 or 31 or 32 or 33 or 34 or 35	37740
37	exp Thromboembolism/ or thromboembolism.mp.	47359
38	(adverse effects or poisoning or toxicity or chemically induced or contraindications or complications).fs.	2846319
39	(adverse adj2 (effect or effects or reaction or reactions or event or events or outcomes or outcome)).mp. [mp=title, original title, abstract, name of substance word, subject heading word, unique identifier]	179933
40	(safe or safety or side-effect* or undesirable effect* or treatment emergent or tolerability or toxicity).mp. [mp=title, original title, abstract, name of substance word, subject heading word, unique identifier]	675202
41	37 or 38 or 39 or 40	3311276
42	10 and 36 and 41	280

ESA harms – search strategy, continued

Database(s):EBM Reviews - Cochrane Central Register of Controlled Trials 4th Quarter 2010
Date searched: 11/15/10

#	Searches	Results
1	anemia.mp. or exp Anemia/c	4561
2	anaemia.mp.	985
3	1 or 2	5004
4	cardiac failure.mp. or exp Heart Failure/	4150
5	chf.mp.	1152
6	congestive heart failure.mp.	2523
7	coronary heart disease.mp. or exp Coronary Disease/	9300
8	ischemic heart disease.mp. or exp Myocardial Ischemia/	17485
9	4 or 5 or 6 or 7 or 8	23230
10	3 and 9	96
11	anti-anaemi*.mp. [mp=title, original title, abstract, mesh headings, heading words, keyword]	0
12	antianaemi*.mp. [mp=title, original title, abstract, mesh headings, heading words, keyword]	1
13	antianemi*.mp. [mp=title, original title, abstract, mesh headings, heading words, keyword]	16
14	anti-anemi*.mp. [mp=title, original title, abstract, mesh headings, heading words, keyword]	5
15	aranesp.mp. [mp=title, original title, abstract, mesh headings, heading words, keyword]	25
16	exp Erythropoietin/ or darbepoetin.mp.	1291
17	darbepoietin.mp.	9
18	darbopoetin.mp. [mp=title, original title, abstract, mesh headings, heading words, keyword]	9
19	epo.mp. [mp=title, original title, abstract, mesh headings, heading words, keyword]	602
20	epoetin.mp. [mp=title, original title, abstract, mesh headings, heading words, keyword]	603
21	epogen.mp. [mp=title, original title, abstract, mesh headings, heading words, keyword]	2
22	epoietin.mp. [mp=title, original title, abstract, mesh headings, heading words, keyword]	18
23	eprex.mp. [mp=title, original title, abstract, mesh headings, heading words, keyword]	22
24	erythropoesis.mp. [mp=title, original title, abstract, mesh headings, heading words, keyword]	5
25	erythropoetin.mp. [mp=title, original title, abstract, mesh headings, heading words, keyword]	32
26	erythropoiesis.mp. [mp=title, original title, abstract, mesh headings, heading words, keyword]	449
27	erythropoietin.mp. [mp=title, original title, abstract, mesh headings, heading words, keyword]	1903

28	ESA.mp. [mp=title, original title, abstract, mesh headings, heading words, keyword]	51
29	ESAs.mp. [mp=title, original title, abstract, mesh headings, heading words, keyword]	18
30	hematinics.mp. [mp=title, original title, abstract, mesh headings, heading words, keyword]	398
31	neorecormon.mp. [mp=title, original title, abstract, mesh headings, heading words, keyword]	19
32	nesp.mp. [mp=title, original title, abstract, mesh headings, heading words, keyword]	23
33	procrit.mp. [mp=title, original title, abstract, mesh headings, heading words, keyword]	13
34	recormon.mp. [mp=title, original title, abstract, mesh headings, heading words, keyword]	7
35	Erythropoiesis-stimulating agent.mp. [mp=title, original title, abstract, mesh headings, heading words, keyword]	28
36	11 or 12 or 13 or 14 or 15 or 16 or 17 or 18 or 19 or 20 or 21 or 22 or 23 or 24 or 25 or 26 or 27 or 28 or 29 or 30 or 31 or 32 or 33 or 34 or 35	2764
37	exp Thromboembolism/ or thromboembolism.mp.	2067
38	(adverse adj2 (effect or effects or reaction or reactions or event or events or outcomes or outcome)).mp.	48156
39	(safe or safety or side-effect* or undesirable effect* or treatment emergent or tolerability or toxicity).mp.	95206
40	37 or 38 or 39	114226
41	10 and 36 and 40	10

ESA harms – search strategy, continued
Database: **EMBASE**
Date searched: 11/15/10

#	Query	Results
11	#7 AND #10	412
10	#8 OR #9	1154469
9	safe OR 'safety'/exp OR 'side effect$' OR undesirable AND effect$ OR treatment AND emergent OR tolerability OR 'toxicity'/exp OR (adverse AND adj2 AND (effect OR effects OR reaction OR reactions OR event OR events OR outcome OR outcomes)) AND [embase]/lim	432305
8	'complication'/exp OR 'side effect'/exp OR 'adverse drug reaction'/exp OR 'drug toxicity'/exp	899447
7	#5 AND #6	1015
6	'anti anami$' OR antianaemi$ OR antianemi$ AND o$r AND 'anti anemi$' OR 'aranesp'/exp OR 'darbepoetin'/exp OR 'darbepoietin'/exp OR 'darbopoetin'/exp OR epo OR 'epoetin'/exp OR 'epogen'/exp OR 'epoietin'/exp OR 'eprex'/exp OR 'erythopoiesis stimulating' AND agents OR erythropoesis OR erythropoetin OR 'erythropoiesis'/exp OR 'erythropoietin'/exp OR esa OR esas OR 'hematinics'/exp OR 'neorecormon'/exp OR 'nesp'/exp OR 'procrit'/exp OR 'recormon'/exp OR rheupo AND [embase]/lim	70423
5	#1 AND #4	5587
4	#2 OR #3	376323
3	'heart failure'/exp OR 'coronary artery disease'/exp	352502
2	cardiac AND failure OR chf OR congestive AND 'heart'/exp AND failure OR coronary AND 'heart'/exp AND 'disease'/exp OR ischemic AND 'heart'/exp AND 'disease'/exp AND [embase]/lim	43081
1	'anemia'/exp AND [embase]/lim	141383

Iron benefits and harms

Database(s):**Ovid MEDLINE® and Ovid OLDMEDLINE®** 1947 to November Week 1 2010, **Ovid MEDLINE® In-Process & Other Non-Indexed Citations** November 11, 2010

#	Searches	Results
1	anemia.mp. or exp Anemia/	149879
2	anaemia.mp.	22339
3	1 or 2	157901
4	cardiac failure.mp. or exp Heart Failure/	77416
5	chf.mp.	8843
6	congestive heart failure.mp.	28353
7	coronary heart disease.mp. or exp Coronary Disease/	177123
8	ischemic heart disease.mp. or exp Myocardial Ischemia/	321932
9	4 or 5 or 6 or 7 or 8	407842
10	3 and 9	2677
11	exp Iron/ or iron.mp.	133944
12	ferric.mp.	18656
13	ferrous.mp.	12391
14	11 or 12 or 13	145012
15	10 and 14	400

Iron benefits and harms – search strategy, continued

Database(s):**EBM Reviews - Cochrane Central Register of Controlled Trials** 4th Quarter 2010
Date searched: 11/15/10

#	Searches	Results
1	anemia.mp. or exp Anemia/	4561
2	anaemia.mp.	985
3	1 or 2	5004
4	cardiac failure.mp. or exp Heart Failure/	4150
5	chf.mp.	1152
6	congestive heart failure.mp.	2523
7	coronary heart disease.mp. or exp Coronary Disease/	9300
8	ischemic heart disease.mp. or exp Myocardial Ischemia/	17485
9	4 or 5 or 6 or 7 or 8	23230
10	3 and 9	96
11	exp Iron/ or iron.mp.	3384
12	ferric.mp.	365
13	ferrous.mp.	604
14	11 or 12 or 13	3566
15	10 and 14	24

Iron benefits and harms – search strategy, continued

Database: **EMBASE**

Date searched: 11/15/10

#	Query	Results
11	#5 AND #10	593
10	#8 OR #9	112969
9	ferric OR ferrous OR 'iron'/exp AND [embase]/lim	85359
8	'iron'/exp	88060
5	#1 AND #4	5587
4	#2 OR #3	376323
3	'heart failure'/exp OR 'coronary artery disease'/exp	352502
2	cardiac AND failure OR chf OR congestive AND 'heart'/exp AND failure OR coronary AND 'heart'/exp AND 'disease'/exp OR ischemic AND 'heart'/exp AND 'disease'/exp AND [embase]/lim	43081
1	'anemia'/exp AND [embase]/lim	141383

RBC transfusion benefits and harms – search strategy

Database(s):**Ovid MEDLINE® and Ovid OLDMEDLINE®** 1947 to November Week 1 2010,
Ovid MEDLINE® In-Process & Other Non-Indexed Citations November 11, 2010

Date searched: 11/12/10

#	Searches	Results
1	anemia.mp. or exp Anemia/	149879
2	anaemia.mp.	22339
3	1 or 2	157901
4	cardiac failure.mp. or exp Heart Failure/	77416
5	chf.mp.	8843
6	congestive heart failure.mp.	28353
7	coronary heart disease.mp. or exp Coronary Disease/	177123
8	ischemic heart disease.mp. or exp Myocardial Ischemia/	321932
9	4 or 5 or 6 or 7 or 8	407842
10	3 and 9	2677
11	red blood cell transfusion.mp. or exp Erythrocyte Transfusion/	5368
12	10 and 11	46

RBC transfusion benefits and harms – search strategy continued

Database(s):**EBM Reviews - Cochrane Central Register of Controlled Trials** 4th Quarter 2010

Date searched: 11/12/10

#	Searches	Results
1	anemia.mp. or exp Anemia/	4561
2	anaemia.mp.	985
3	1 or 2	5004
4	cardiac failure.mp. or exp Heart Failure/	4150
5	chf.mp.	1152
6	congestive heart failure.mp.	2523
7	coronary heart disease.mp. or exp Coronary Disease/	9300
8	ischemic heart disease.mp. or exp Myocardial Ischemia/	17485
9	4 or 5 or 6 or 7 or 8	23230
10	3 and 9	96
11	red blood cell transfusion.mp. or exp Erythrocyte Transfusion/	360
12	10 and 11	6

RBC transfusion benefits and harms – search strategy continued
Database(s):**EMBASE**
Date searched: 11/12/10

#	Query	Results
7	#5 AND #6	205
6	'erythrocyte transfusion'/exp	8844
5	#1 AND #4	5587
4	#2 OR #3	376323
3	'heart failure'/exp OR 'coronary artery disease'/exp	352502
2	cardiac AND failure OR chf OR congestive AND 'heart'/exp AND failure OR coronary AND 'heart'/exp AND 'disease'/exp OR ischemic AND 'heart'/exp AND 'disease'/exp AND [embase]/lim	43081
1	'anemia'/exp AND [embase]/lim	141383

Hemoglobin threshold – search strategy
Database(s):**Ovid MEDLINE® and Ovid OLDMEDLINE®** 1947 to November Week 1 2010,
Ovid MEDLINE® In-Process & Other Non-Indexed Citations November 11, 2010

#	Searches	Results
1	(hemoglobin adj3 threshold*).mp. [mp=title, original title, abstract, name of substance word, subject heading word, unique identifier]	75

Hemoglobin threshold – search strategy continued
Database: **EMBASE**
Date searched: 11/12/10

#	Query	Results
7	#5 AND #6	16
6	threshold AND 'hemoglobin'/exp AND [embase]/lim	972
5	#1 AND #4	5587
4	#2 OR #3	376323
3	'heart failure'/exp OR 'coronary artery disease'/exp	352502
2	cardiac AND failure OR chf OR congestive AND 'heart'/exp AND failure OR coronary AND 'heart'/exp AND 'disease'/exp OR ischemic AND 'heart'/exp AND 'disease'/exp AND [embase]/lim	43081
1	'anemia'/exp AND [embase]/lim	141383

Hemoglobin threshold – search strategy continued
Database(s):**EBM Reviews - Cochrane Central Register of Controlled Trials** 4th Quarter 2010
Date searched: 11/12/10

#	Searches	Results
1	(hemoglobin adj3 threshold*).mp. [mp=title, original title, abstract, mesh headings, heading words, keyword]	14

APPENDIX B. INCLUSION/EXCLUSION CRITERIA

1. Is the full text of the article in English?
   Yes..Proceed to #2
   No.. Code **X1**. STOP

2. Does the study population include adult patients with congestive heart failure or coronary heart disease, and anemia or iron deficiency?
   Yes..Proceed to #3
   No... Code X2. Proceed to #8

3. Is the article an intervention study (or a systematic review/meta-analysis of intervention studies) comparing the effects of ESAs, iron, or red blood cell transfusions with usual care or placebo; or an observational study of the effects of red blood cell transfusions?
   Yes..Proceed to #4
   No..Go to #5

4. Does the study report outcomes that include mortality, hospitalization, exercise tolerance, cardiovascular events, quality of life, or adverse effects of treatment?
   Yes...Code I4. Go to #6
   No .... Code X4. Go to #7

5. Is the article an observational study that reports data on the harms of using ESAs or iron?
   Yes...Code I5. Proceed to #6
   No... Code X5. Proceed to #7

6. Does the article describe or analyze the costs of treatment or implementation?
   Yes... Add Code C. STOP
   No...STOP

7. Does the article describe or analyze the costs of treatment or implementation?
   Yes... Add Code C. STOP
   No..Proceed to #8

8. Is the article potentially useful for background, discussion, or reference-mining?
   Yes..Code B. STOP
   No.. STOP

Treatment of Anemia in Patients with Heart Disease: A Systematic Review

APPENDIX C. QUALITY ASSESSMENT TABLES

Appendix C, Table 1. Assessment of methodologic characteristics and risk of bias in randomized controlled trials of ESA therapy in patients with CHF or CHD

Study ID	Was the allocation sequence adequately generated?	Was allocation adequately concealed?	Blinding of participants, personnel and outcome assessors: Was knowledge of the allocated intervention adequately prevented?	Were incomplete outcome data adequately addressed?	Selective outcome reporting: Are reports of the study free of suggestion of selective outcome reporting?	Other sources of bias: Was the study apparently free of other problems that could put it at a high risk of bias?	Summary assessment: risk of bias (Low, Unclear, High)
Bellinghieri, 1994[27]	Unclear	Unclear	No	No	Unclear	No serious baseline imbalances. Randomized, but very little baseline characteristics presented though the baseline gender imbalance raises concerns that groups may not have been equal at baseline.	Overall: high risk of bias
Besarab 1998[26]	Unclear	Unclear	Yes - low risk of bias for mortality outcome, probably low risk of bias for hospitalization, MI outcomes. High risk of bias for physical function outcome given that blinding of participants and outcome assessors is unlikely to have occurred	Low risk of bias - data for all patients enrolled is reported and an intention to treat analysis was done	It is unclear why a composite outcome was chosen. Functional status data were incompletely reported (no comparative data, only that functional status increased with increasing Hct levels) --> high risk of bias for functional status outcomes, but probably low risk of bias for mortality outcome	No serious baseline imbalances between groups.	Overall: low risk of bias
Comin-Colet, 2009[12]	No - high risk of bias - allocation by preference of the participant. Because preference for treatment could be associated with unmeasured confounders such as better self-management skills etc, this is a significant methodologic limitation which threatens the validity of the results.	No	No - high risk of bias for subjective outcomes	Yes	Unclear	No serious baseline imbalances between groups	Overall: high risk of bias
Ghali, 2008[19]	Yes	Yes	Yes	Yes	Unclear	No serious baseline imbalances between groups	Overall: low risk of bias
Kourea, 2008[17]	Unclear	Unclear	Yes - though single blind, it was placebo controlled and evaluation of QOL and depression surveys was done by blinded personnel	Yes	Unclear	No serious baseline imbalances between groups	Overall: Unclear risk of bias

Treatment of Anemia in Patients with Heart Disease: A Systematic Review

Study ID	Was the allocation sequence adequately generated?	Was allocation adequately concealed?	Blinding of participants, personnel and outcome assessors: Was knowledge of the allocated intervention adequately prevented?	Were incomplete outcome data adequately addressed?	Selective outcome reporting: Are reports of the study free of suggestion of selective outcome reporting?	Other sources of bias: Was the study apparently free of other problems that could put it at a high risk of bias?	Summary assessment: risk of bias (Low, Unclear, High)
Mancini, 2003[24]	Unclear	Unclear	Personnel and outcome assessors were not blinded. High risk of bias especially for QOL outcomes	Yes, though no ITT done, only 3 patients did not complete treatment	No - high risk of bias - no protocol available. The QOL outcome is not completely reported - no actual values, only that x % "improved" and the definition of improvement is not provided.	No serious baseline imbalances between groups	Overall: high risk of bias
Palazzuoli, 2006[28]	Unclear	Unclear	Yes	Yes	Unclear	No serious baseline imbalances between groups. It is unclear if there is any overlap between patients in this study and Palazzuoli 2009 - if so, then possible multiple publication bias	Overall: Unclear risk of bias, but duplicates Palazzuoli 2007 results
Palazzuoli, 2007[21]	Unclear	Unclear	No (for 12 month outcomes) - high risk of bias for 12 month outcomes such as NYHA class. Blinding stopped after 4 month mark.	No - high risk of bias. Not clear that ITT done. Nowhere in the results is the denominator actually reported so it is unclear what the final n was used to calculate results.	No - no protocol available. The study includes 12 month NYHA scores as an outcome, but there are no objective measures of exercise duration which one might expect as another secondary outcome measure.	No serious baseline imbalances between groups. It is unclear if there is any overlap between patients in this study and Palazzuoli 2009 - if so, then possible multiple publication bias	Overall: high risk of bias. Duplicates Palazzuoli 2006 results with some additions.
Palazzuoli, 2009[15]	Unclear	Unclear	Blinding of personnel and outcome assessors is unclear past the 4 month mark after which intervention drug was continued, but the control group saline injections were discontinued. This could create high risk of bias for outcomes such as NYHA class.	No - high risk of bias. No ITT done. 7 of 58 enrolled patients did not make it to f/u and though outcomes are briefly and incompletely described for these patients they are not included in analyses. Additionally, only 48 of the 58 pts were included in the hospitalization outcome and the reasons for the discrepant numbers are not explained.	No - high risk of bias. No protocol available. The incomplete reporting of all enrolled patients raises suspicion that not all outcomes were reported. Further, there are signals from within paper that this is so (eg - edema development was a secondary end point but is not reported in results). Other secondary end points are incompletely described ("no significant changes in myocardial events was seen")	No serious baseline imbalances between groups.	Overall: high risk of bias
Parissis, 2008[18]	Yes	Unclear	Yes - single blind. Personnel not blinded, but outcome assessors were	Yes	Unclear	No serious baseline imbalances between groups. It is unclear if there is any overlap between patients in this study and Parissis 2009 – if so, then possible multiple publication bias	Overall: low risk of bias

Treatment of Anemia in Patients with Heart Disease: A Systematic Review

Study ID	Was the allocation sequence adequately generated?	Was allocation adequately concealed?	Blinding of participants, personnel and outcome assessors: Was knowledge of the allocated intervention adequately prevented?	Were incomplete outcome data adequately addressed?	Selective outcome reporting: Are reports of the study free of suggestion of selective outcome reporting?	Other sources of bias: Was the study apparently free of other problems that could put it at a high risk of bias?	Summary assessment: risk of bias (Low, Unclear, High)
Parissis, 2009[16]	Yes	Unclear	Yes - single blind. Personnel not blinded but outcome assessors were	Yes	Unclear	No serious baseline imbalances between groups. It is unclear if there is any overlap between patients in this study and Parissis 2008 - if so, then possible multiple publication bias	Overall: low risk of bias
Pfeffer, 2009[14]	Yes	Unclear	Yes	Yes - 13% attrition, but equally balanced between two groups	Unclear	No serious baseline imbalances between groups	Overall: low risk of bias
Ponikowski, 2007[23]	Yes	Yes	Yes	Yes	Unclear	No serious baseline imbalances between groups Some evidence of spin: QOL assessed by three measures and improvement seen only in one measure, not the other two, yet conclusions suggest ESA improved health related quality of life	Overall: low risk of bias
Silverberg, 2001[25]	Unclear	No "Randomization… not done in a blinded fashion"	No	Unclear - Nowhere in the results is the denominator actually reported so it is unclear what the final n was used to calculate results.	Unclear	No serious baseline imbalances between groups	Overall: high risk of bias
Van Veldhuisen, 2007[22]	Yes	Yes	Yes	Yes	Unclear	No serious baseline imbalances between groups	Overall: low risk of bias

Appendix C, Table 2. Assessment of methodologic characteristics and risk of bias in randomized controlled trials of RBC transfusion for anemia in patients with CHF or CHD

Study ID	Was the allocation sequence adequately generated?	Was allocation adequately concealed?	Blinding of participants, personnel and outcome assessors: Was knowledge of the allocated intervention adequately prevented?	Were incomplete outcome data adequately addressed?	Are reports of the study free of suggestion of selective outcome reporting?	Other sources of bias: Was the study apparently free of other problems that could put it at a high risk of bias?	Summary assessment: risk of bias (Low, Unclear, High)
Bracey, 1999[65]	Unclear: last digit of HR# determined group assignment	Unclear, concealment method not described	Study not described as blinded.	Yes	Yes	No serious baseline imbalances between groups.	Overall: Unclear risk of bias
Bush, 1997[67]	Unclear: randomization method not specified	Yes (sealed envelopes)	Study not described as blinded. Surgeons and anesthesiologists were not blinded.	Yes	Yes	No serious baseline imbalances between groups.	Overall: Low risk of bias
Carson, 1998[68]	Yes: automated telephone-response system at a separate research institute.	Yes: automated telephone-response system at a separate research institute.	Outcome assessors were blinded; blinding was not otherwise specified for patients or care personnel.	Yes	Yes	No serious baseline imbalances between groups.	Overall: Low risk of bias
Carson, 2009[69]	Unclear: randomization method not described (abstract only)	Not described (abstract only)	Not described (abstract only)	Not described (abstract only)	Yes	No serious baseline imbalances between groups.	Overall: Probably low; study is based on the pilot trial above (Carson 1998)
Cooper, 2011[40] CRIT trial	Unclear: randomization method not specified	Yes (opaque envelopes)	No: "Blinding of treatment assignment was not feasible"	Yes; 6.7% loss to follow-up	Yes	More smokers in conservative group (10% v 33%); more diabetes in liberal group (81% v 54%); P-values not specified.	Overall: Low risk of bias
Hajjar, 2010[66]	Yes (random numbers table)	Yes (opaque envelopes)	Patient and outcome assessors were blinded to group assignment. Anesthesiologist and ICU health care workers were not blinded.	Yes	Yes	No serious baseline imbalances between groups.	Overall: Low risk of bias
Hebert, 2001[39] TRICC trial	Unclear: randomization method not specified	Unclear, concealment method not described	Outcome assessors were blinded; care personnel were not blinded; patient blinding not specified.	Yes	Yes	No serious baseline imbalances between groups.	Overall: Low risk of bias
Johnson, 1992[64]	Yes (random numbers table)	Unclear, concealment method not described	Surgeons and anesthesiologists were blinded until patient in ICU. Blinding of outcome assessor and patient not specified.	Yes. No in-hospital deaths occurred.	Yes	No serious baseline imbalances between groups.	Overall: Low risk of bias
Weisel, 1984[63]	Unclear: randomization method not specified	Unclear, concealment method not described	Use of blinding was not stated.	Yes	Yes	No serious baseline imbalances between groups.	Overall: Low risk of bias

71

Appendix C, Table 3. Assessment of methodologic characteristics and risk of bias in observational studies of RBC transfusions for anemia in patients with CHD/CHF, stratified by patient population

Author Year	Non-biased selection?	High overall loss to follow-up or differential loss to follow-up?	Outcomes pre-specified and defined?	Ascertainment techniques adequately described?	Non-biased and adequate ascertainment methods?	Statistical analysis of potential confounders?			Comments	Adequate duration of follow-up?
						Propensity matching	Account for bleeding	Account for timing of transfusion		
Percutaneous Coronary Intervention										
Chase, 2008[48] Multicenter Canada	Yes	No	Yes	Yes	Yes	Yes	No	No	Multivariate analysis did not account for some important confounders such as CHF	30 day and 1 year
Doyle, 2008[47] Mayo clinic USA	Yes	Not reported	Yes	No. Hospital complication registry but method of follow-up not stated	Not reported	No	No	No	Confounders not reported	Unclear, 30 day mortality reported, but graphs show 5-6 year mortality trends.
Jani, 2007[49]	Yes	No	Yes	Yes	Yes	Yes	Yes	No		Yes
Jolicoeur, 2009[50]	Yes	No	Yes	Yes	Yes	Yes	Yes	Yes		Yes
Kim, 2007[45] Single center USA	Yes	No	Yes	Yes	Yes	Yes	Yes	No		1 year
Kinnaird, 2003[44] Single center USA	Yes	Probably No. Lost 14%. Difference in loss between groups not reported.	Yes	Yes	Yes	No	Yes	No		1 year
Maluenda, 2009[36] Single Institution USA	Yes	Not reported	Yes	Yes	Probably yes	No	Yes	No		30 days and 1 year.
Maluenda, 2009[37]	Unknown. Abstract only reports # of charts reviewed. Probably yes as is likely same cohort as above.	Not reported	Yes.	No.	Probably yes as likely is same registry as above. But unknown based on this abstract.				Abstract only, may be same population as other Maluenda reference	1 year
Maluenda, 2009[38]	Unknown Abstract only reports # of charts reviewed. Probably yes as is likely same cohort as above.	Not reported	Yes	No.	Probably yes as likely is same registry as above. But unknown based on this abstract.				Abstract only, may be same population as other Maluenda reference	1 year

Treatment of Anemia in Patients with Heart Disease: A Systematic Review

Author Year	Non-biased selection?	High overall loss to follow-up or differential loss to follow-up?	Outcomes pre-specified and defined?	Ascertainment techniques adequately described?	Non-biased and adequate ascertainment methods?	Statistical analysis of potential confounders?				Adequate duration of follow-up?
						Propensity matching	Account for bleeding	Account for timing of transfusion	Comments	
Nikolsky, 2009[51]	Yes	No	Yes	Yes	Yes	Yes	Yes	No		Yes
Yatskar, 2007[46] Multicenter USA	Yes	No	Yes	Mostly yes. NHLBI registry. Telephone follow-up. But unclear why they looked at "Hematoma Related Transfusion" rather than transfusion.	Probably yes. Again, didn't look at transfusions, only hematoma related transfusions.	No	No – only examined transfusions for hematoma, but not for other causes or for transfusion without bleeding.	No	Confounders not reported and appears a number of important confounders were probably not accounted for	1 year

Acute Coronary Syndrome/Acute MI

Author Year	Non-biased selection?	High overall loss to follow-up or differential loss to follow-up?	Outcomes pre-specified and defined?	Ascertainment techniques adequately described?	Non-biased and adequate ascertainment methods?	Propensity matching	Account for bleeding	Account for timing of transfusion	Comments	Adequate duration of follow-up?
Aggarwal, 2011[60]	Partly - unclear whether transfusion administration was prospectively collected data for all potentially eligible patients.	No	Yes	No, but primary outcome was in-hospital death.	Yes, probably	No	Yes	No		Yes
Alexander, 2008[55]	Yes	No	Yes	Yes	Yes	No	No	No		Yes
Aronson, 2008[58]	Yes	Not reported	Yes	Yes	Unclear if investigators doing chart review on repeat admissions were blinded to whether patient had transfusion.	Yes	No	No		Yes
Rao, 2004[52]	Yes	No	Yes	Yes	Yes	Yes	Yes	Yes		Yes
Sabatine, 2005[57]	Yes	No	Yes	Yes	Yes	No	Yes	No		Yes
Shishehbor, 2009[56]	Yes	No	Yes	Yes	Yes	Yes	Yes	Yes	Also conducted sensitivity analyses to determine impact of "hidden" biases and found there would have to be "enormous" hidden biases to account for results	Yes
Singla, 2007[54]	Yes	No	Yes	Yes	No, 30 day event rates limited to VA hospitals only.	No	No	No		Yes

Treatment of Anemia in Patients with Heart Disease: A Systematic Review

Author Year	Non-biased selection?	High overall loss to follow-up or differential loss to follow-up?	Outcomes pre-specified and defined?	Ascertainment techniques adequately described?	Non-biased and adequate ascertainment methods?	Statistical analysis of potential confounders?			Comments	Adequate duration of follow-up?
						Propensity matching	Account for bleeding	Account for timing of transfusion		
Wu, 2001[59]	Yes	No, probably - primary outcome 30 D mortality assessed using Medicare Enrollment database, but proportion with complete vital status at 30 D unclear.	Yes	Yes	Yes, probably.	Yes	No	Partly – conducted additional analysis excluding patients who died within two days of admission.	Unclear how well transfusion administration was captured by claims data.	Yes
Yang, 2005[53]	Yes	Unclear - CRUSADE QI initiative relies on retrospective chart review.	Yes	No	No - in-hospital outcomes only, unclear whether post-discharge deaths were accounted for.	No	No	No		No
Congestive Heart Failure										
Garty, 2009[61]	Yes	No	Yes	Yes	Yes	Yes	No	No		Yes
Kao, 2011[62]	Yes	No	Yes	Yes	Yes	No	No	No		Yes
Critical Illness										
Hebert, 1997[71]	Unclear - consecutive patients, but 40% were retrospectively identified and patient identification methods not well-described.	Unclear	Yes	No	Unclear	No	No	No		Yes
Surgery										
Bursi, 2009[41]	Yes	Unclear - number of patients with complete 30 day survival information not reported	Yes	Partly	Partly - 30 day mortality assessed through review of death certificates and phone interviews, but not clear they looked at death registries	Yes	Yes	Yes		Yes
Carson, 1998[81]	Yes	No	Yes	Yes	Yes	Yes	Yes	Unclear		Yes
Glance, 2011[70]	Yes	No	Yes	Yes	Yes	Yes	No	No	Did not account for post-operative transfusions.	Yes

74

APPENDIX D. PEER REVIEW COMMENTS AND RESPONSES

Reviewer	Comment	Response
Question 1: Are the objectives, scope, and methods for this review clearly described?		
1	No: I am worried about a few things in the current iteration of the review: 1) defining the population upfront; 2) defining the outcomes upfront; 3) justification of the inclusion of observational data. Defining the population – the document refers to patients with "CHF" and "CHD" but does not drill down and define these. CHF can include those with asymptomatic low LVEF or those with symptoms of CHF but with normal LVEF. Similarly, CHD can include acute coronary syndrome, PCI, or those with stable angina. I think these clinical entities need to be defined upfront.	We've clarified these definitions in the "study selection" section of Methods. The entities had been defined (fairly broadly) up front, but we agree this was not well-reported in the manuscript.
1	If the studies are heterogeneous in their inclusion of these populations, then this should be specifically mentioned.	We've added more detail to the "data abstraction" section of Methods to clarify that we've collected and reported the clinical characteristics of study populations. We also added a sentence to the second paragraph of Discussion clarifying that most ESA studies were in patients with systolic heart failure. The applicability of the evidence review findings to various patient populations is also further delineated in the GRADE table, and in the clinical applications section.
1	Also, why examine non-anemic patients with iron deficiency if the primary purpose is to study the treatment of anemia?	Clarified this in "study selection" section.
1	Defining the outcomes – the document examines several outcomes but no justification is provided for why they were chosen.	Clarified that we are defining "health outcome" as those that are patient-centered and apparent to the patient (in contrast to intermediate physiologic outcomes). The list of outcomes was discussed with and approved by the Technical Expert Panel during the topic development phase.
1	Justification of observational data – on pages 7 and 8, there is a section on Study Quality, and the answers to all of the questions posed would result in observational data being "low quality." This is entirely justified, but there are other ways to evaluate observational data like the appropriateness and robustness of the statistical methods. The authors should consider including some measure of observational data quality.	We've added a table describing the methodologic characteristics of each of the observational studies. We've added the quality assessment description to "study quality" section of Methods.
2	Agree with adding ortho surgery data as large RCT recently completed.	The data had not been available, but we will include if enough data available.
3	Yes.	
Question 2: Is there any indication of bias in our synthesis of the evidence?		
1	The only bias is in the observational studies that are included (see above).	Noted and discussed above.
2	Seemed to be more pro-ESA than the data supports	Noted
3	No.	
Question 3: Are there any published or unpublished studies that we may have overlooked?		
1	No.	Noted.
2	The ortho FOCUS trial	See comment 5 rows below regarding the FOCUS trial.
3	No.	Noted.

Treatment of Anemia in Patients with Heart Disease: A Systematic Review

Reviewer	Comment	Response
Question 4:	*Please write additional suggestions or comments below. If applicable, please indicate the page and line numbers from the draft report.*	
1	The section on iron therapy doesn't seem to have a summary of what the overall findings are. This would be helpful.	Thanks – yes, an accidental omission – this was added to the beginning of the iron section.
1	Page 39 – MINT is an ongoing trial and likely will not be published for several years. There is a trial that has been presented called FOCUS that will be published soon. (see http://www.theheart.org/article/1024017.do for a report of the presented results).	Thanks for the clarification. The results were amended accordingly. We report the FOCUS results available in an abstract and acknowledge the full document has yet to be published.
1	Page 40 – an important distinction between the Wu study and the Rao study are that Wu looked at *baseline* anemia while Rao examined the lowest hct value occurring during hospitalization. In addition, patients with active bleeding were excluded from the Wu study.	We've clarified these distinctions in this section of the discussion.
1	The section on Clinical Applications should be more prescriptive (see below). It's tough to actually get at what the recommendation is because it is obscured a bit by more description of the data.	We've stopped short of providing prescriptive recommendations of what should and should not be done intentionally as we'd feel more comfortable developing clinical recommendations in conjunction with our stakeholders/clinical partners.
2	Page 2- need to give number of paper rejected	Thank you – we had accidentally omitted this from the executive summary.
2	Page 2 – ESA – to me the evidence is clear that ESA are associated with harm and not "may be". This is especially true in diabetic patients	The harm of targeting near-normal hemoglobin, especially in diabetic patients, seems clear after trials like TREAT, but these were not exclusively focused on treatment of anemic heart disease patients. The harms of using ESAs in heart disease populations are not as well elucidated. The language is meant to reflect this uncertainty and the fact that it most closely applies to those with chronic kidney disease. However, we did change the language to be a bit more direct (changed "possibility" to "finding," and "may be" to "is".
2	Page 9 – the hematocrit to hemoglobin correction of 10:1 makes no sense – the Hbg:Hct is 1:3 roughly.	Thank you – this was a typo – corrected.
2	Page 12 – again I think the case ESA cause harm is proven	Please see response to page 2 comment above.
2	Page 16 – would strongly disagree that 6MWT is not influence by blinding – reams of data in the sports medicine literature supports placebo effect!	Thank you – yes, we had mis-stated this. Meant to say lack of personnel blinding alone, given that outcome assessors were blinded, shouldn't carry high risk of bias for these outcomes. Patients were blinded, and control patients received placebo injections. We've clarified this in the table.
2	Page 21- is there data to support the notion that longer use of ESA is associated with greater harm?	It would be hard to determine this from the studies. The two studies mentioned with long follow-up periods also differed in patient population and treatment from the other smaller, shorter duration ESA trials. The mortality curves in Besarab did begin to separate several months into treatment and continued to diverge 1-2 years into treatment.
2	Page 26 – any data for increased risk of cancer? Was suggested in TRICK study and certainly seen in the oncology trials….	No, not that was reported in these trials. Of note, many excluded patients with malignancy.
2	Page 26 – just a comment – are the ongoing trials even ethical given what we know about high Hct goals and bad outcomes with ESA…	Interesting point, but outside the scope of our review. It is a different patient population.

Reviewer	Comment	Response
2	Page 29 – Although old, I have found the discussion in this paper the best framework for understanding the complex interplay of transfusions for cardiac disease: *Prudent strategies for elective red blood cell transfusion. Welch HG, Meehan KR, Goodnough LT. Ann Intern Med. 1992 Mar 1;116(5):393-402*	Thanks for this suggestion.
2	Page 32 – any suggestion of confounder of ACS management and risk of transfusion – i.e. if more patients have PCI that did worse with more transfusions??	One of the main confounders would be risk of bleeding associated with management – either procedural or med-related. Not all studies accounted for bleeding, but some did and we've added a table clarifying some of the methodologic characteristics of observational transfusion studies, including whether or not they accounted for bleeding complications.
2	Page 38 – the FDA ESA recommendation is even more aggressive than stated: *In controlled trials with CKD patients, patients experienced greater risks for death, serious adverse cardiovascular reactions, and stroke when administered ESAs to target a hemoglobin level of greater than 11 g/dL.* *No trial has identified a hemoglobin target level, ESA dose, or dosing strategy that does not increase these risks.* *ESA labels now recommend:* *For patients with CKD, consider starting ESA treatment when the hemoglobin level is less than 10 g/dL. This advice does not define how far below 10 g/dL is appropriate for an individual to initiate. This advice also does not recommend that the goal is to achieve a hemoglobin of 10 g/dL or a hemoglobin above 10 g/dL. Individualize dosing and use the lowest dose of ESA sufficient to reduce the need for red blood cell transfusions. Adjust dosing as appropriate.*	Agree. We've tried to clarify the language further by inserting the phrase "if they are to be used at all".
2	Page 39: - the "10/30" was based on an off the cuff recommendation by a Mayo Anesthesiologist in WWII (Vox Sang. 2010 Jan;98(1):2-11)	Thank you. We've inserted this reference.
2	Page 40 – given that most ACS patients in the USA get PCI should transfusions be proscribed in them for hbg > 8-9??	This is a question for policy- and guideline-makers. The data summarized here are still largely of poor quality because it is mostly observational data.
2	Page 41 – The person with the ferritin of 50 is truly iron deficiency and needs some form of iron replacement - also needs a GI work-up – maybe a ferritin of 123 would make the point better	We felt the data was not as strong for patients with ferritin > 100. The Anker study included patients with higher ferritins, but most had ferritin well below 100 and the applicability of the results of this IV iron trial are strongest for patients with low ferritins.
2	Page 42 – I though the trial for ESA for STEMI was distinctly negative - *JAMA. 2011 May 11;305(18):1863-72. Intravenous erythropoietin in patients with ST-segment elevation myocardial infarction: REVEAL: a randomized controlled trial. Najjar SS, Rao SV, Melloni C, Raman SV, Povsic TJ, Melton L, Barsness GW, Prather K, Heitner JF, Kilaru R, Gruberg L, Hasselblad V, Greenbaum AB, Patel M, Kim RJ, Talan M, Ferrucci L, Longo DL, Lakatta EG, Harrington RA; REVEAL Investigators.* – also stroke - *Stroke. 2009 Dec;40(12):e647-56*	This and 2 other recent trials examined one-time high-dose ESA use in ACS patients but these were not focused on treatment of anemic patients. As such, they fell outside of the scope of our review. Inclusion of the statement alluding to these studies in our discussion is probably confusing and we've deleted it.

Reviewer	Comment	Response
3	Overall excellent review. The "emerging themes" concept is great as it does not leave the reader hanging in his/her approach to the individual patient. Love the way you broke out the high quality studies in fig 3 and 4.	Noted. Thanks.
3	On page 2- need to fill in # of studies rejected. Page 11- first box on right needs the N filled in.	Done.
3	We can develop practice guidelines around this but would not promulgate quality measures just yet.	Noted.
4	Overall –very readable, a seemingly transparent, honest assessment of the literature leaving this reader confident in the findings and the interpretations.	Noted.
4	Never easy to give weight to benefits and harms, or benefits versus harms, the problem was not clearly resolved in this analysis. I've no suggestions and in general thought the balance reached by the authors was reasonable.	Noted.
4	Except for the one ongoing study of 80 patients, all (or the vast, vast majority) patients apparently had recognized systolic dysfunction. In some CHF series, up to half have normal ejection fractions. . While I can't think why this would group would fare differently with treatments for anemia, available studies don't apply. . In some clinical trials evaluating arrhythmia patients, a clinical history of CHF was a more powerful predictor of outcome than ejection fraction measurements.	Agree. We've added statements to the ESA "summary" paragraph in results, the ESA discussion, and the Future studies sections clarifying that this evidence base applies most directly to those with reduced systolic function.
4	No data on influence of very common and potentially important contributors to outcomes….smoking, lung disease, cardiovascular medications, arrhythmias (particularly atrial fibrillation), others….	We limited the ESA and iron sections to trials only. We examined each trial for important baseline differences, though most were adequately randomized. This is more of an issue for the observational transfusion studies and we have evaluated the methodologic characteristics – including accounting for important confounders – of these studies.
Question 5: Are there any clinical performance measures, programs, quality improvement measures, patient care services, or conferences that will be directly affected by this report? If so, please provide detail.		
1	Absolutely. The use of blood is high in the VA system as is the use of ESAs. By providing this document, the use of these therapies with limited benefit should be curbed resulting in safer care for veterans at lower cost.	Noted.
2	Yes – this report has wide implications for multiple areas of care	Noted.
3	Each individual institution/system will need to assess its use of ESA's, iron and transfusions in these populations.	Noted.
Question 6. Please provide any recommendations on how this report can be revised to more directly address or assist implementation needs.		
1	I think the section on Clinical Applications should be more prescriptive. Also the clinical scenarios are a bit strange. I would prefer to see broader categories, or if this is too difficult, a table with the first column being the clinical situation and the subsequent columns addressing ESAs, Iron, and Blood transfusion. The cells then could have a (+), (-), or "Unk" for whether the evidence supports use or if there are no data.	We intended the GRADE table to show the level of evidence in various broad clinical categories for each of the interventions.
2	I think the transfusion part could stand alone as a journal article	Noted.
3	Target not only the cardiology and hospitalist leaders, but the P&T and blood bank chairs at system levels.	Noted.

www.ingramcontent.com/pod-product-compliance
Lightning Source LLC
Chambersburg PA
CBHW081555170526
45166CB00009B/2712